DEMENTIA CARE INSERVICE TRAINING MODULES for LONG-TERM CARE

To my grandmother who was consumed by Alzheimer's disease and continues as a spiritual strength in my life. I dedicate this book to you and all my wonderful memories.

I love you

Lisa Celia

To my unborn son, who is in my present thoughts, who will remind me of my past and who will remember my future.

Jackie Nasso

DEMENTIA CARE INSERVICE TRAINING MODULES for LONG-TERM CARE

Jackie Nasso, RN, BSN, MPA
Lisa Celia, RN, BSN

THOMSON
DELMAR LEARNING

Australia   Brazil   Canada   Mexico   Singapore   Spain   United   Kingdom   United States

THOMSON
DELMAR LEARNING

Dementia Care: InService Training Modules for Long-Term Care
by Jackie Nasso and Lisa Celia

Vice President, Health Care Business Unit:
William Brottmiller

Director of Learning Solutions:
Matthew Kane

Managing Editor:
Marah Bellegarde

Acquisitions Editor:
Matthew Seeley

Product Manager:
Jadin Babin-Kavanaugh

Marketing Director:
Jennifer McAvey

Marketing Manager:
Michele McTighe

Technology Director:
Laurie Davis

Technology Project Coordinator:
Carolyn Fox

Production Director:
Carolyn Miller

Production Manager:
Barbara A. Bullock

Content Project Manager:
Anne Sherman

COPYRIGHT © 2007 by Thomson Delmar Learning, a part of The Thomson Corporation. Thomson, the Star logo, and Delmar Learning are trademarks used herein under license.

Printed in the United States of America
1 2 3 4 5 6 7 XXX 08 07 06

For more information, contact Thomson Delmar Learning, 5 Maxwell Drive, Clifton Park, NY 12065-2919
Or you can visit our Internet site at http://www.delmarlearning.com

ALL RIGHTS RESERVED. No part of this work covered by the copyright hereon may be reproduced or used in any form or by any means—graphic, electronic, or mechanical, including photocopying, recording, taping, Web distribution or information storage and retrieval systems—without the written permission of the publisher.

For permission to use material from this text or product, contact us by
Tel (800) 730-2214
Fax (800) 730-2215
www.thomsonrights.com

Library of Congress Cataloging-in-Publication Data

Nasso, Jackie.
  Dementia care: inservice training modules for long-term care / Jackie Nasso, Lisa Celia
    p. cm.
  Includes bibliographical references.
  ISBN-13: 978-1-4018-9858-8 (pbk.)
  ISBN-10: 1-4018-9858-0 (pbk.)
  1. Dementia—Patients—Long term care—Study and teaching. 2. Dementia—Nursing—Study and teaching. I. Celia, Lisa. II. Title.
  RC521.N37 2007
  616.8'3--dc22

2006015041

NOTICE TO THE READER

Publisher does not warrant or guarantee any of the products described herein or perform any independent analysis in connection with any of the product information contained herein. Publisher does not assume, and expressly disclaims, any obligation to obtain and include information other than that provided to it by the manufacturer.

The reader is expressly warned to consider and adopt all safety precautions that might be indicated by the activities described herein and to avoid all potential hazards. By following the instructions contained herein, the reader willingly assumes all risks in connection with such instructions.

The publisher makes no representations or warranties of any kind, including but not limited to, the warranties of fitness for particular purpose or merchantability, nor are any such representations implied with respect to the material set forth herein, and the publisher takes no responsibility with respect to such material. The publisher shall not be liable for any special, consequential, or exemplary damages resulting, in whole or part, from the readers' use of, or reliance upon, this material.

Contents

Introduction ix

Effective Teaching Strategies xi

Module 1 — Understanding Dementia 1

General Information/Overview • 2
Types of Dementia • 2
The Normal Human Brain • 5
Neurons • 7
Neuron Changes with AD • 7
Effects of AD on Cerebral Function • 8
Factors Increasing the Risk for AD • 10
Signs and Symptoms of Dementia • 12
Diagnostic Evaluation • 14
Diagnosing Alzheimer's Disease • 15
Stage of AD • 16
Treatments for AD • 19
Observation and Reporting • 21
How to Report Changes • 23
Summing Up • 24
Real-Life Scenario • 25
Purpose of the Activity • 26
Handouts and Transparency Masters • 27

Module 2 — Basic Principles of Dementia Care 53

General Information/Overview • 54
Developing a Plan of Care • 54
Behavioral and Memory Interventions • 57
The Communication Process • 59
Common Communication Characteristics among Clients
with Alzheimer's Disease • 60
Communication Abilities Preserved in AD Clients • 61
Behavioral Challenges • 63
Exploring Causes and Solutions to Behavioral Changes • 65
Common Behavioral Symptoms Associated with AD • 66
Basic Principles of Care • 74

v

Summing Up • 76
Real-Life Scenario • 77
Handouts and Transparency Masters • 79

Module 3

Daily Care 95

General Information/Overview • 96
Daily Care • 96
Maintaining Physical Health • 97
Maintaining the Physical Environment • 98
Maintaining a Supportive Social Environment • 99
Bathing • 100
Oral Care • 102
Dressing • 106
Toileting • 108
Incontinence • 108
Urinary Incontinence • 110
Toileting Regimen • 111
Summing Up • 113
Real-Life Scenario • 114
Handouts and Transparency Masters • 116

Module 4

Eating Challenges with Dementia 135

General Information/Overview • 136
Plan of Care • 137
Ideational Apraxia • 139
Maintaining a Supportive Physical Environment • 139
Maintaining a Supportive Social Environment • 141
Eating as an Activity • 142
Observation and Reporting of Feeding Patterns • 143
Eating Challenges • 144
Eating Safety • 146
Signs of Dysphagia • 148
Oral Feedings Versus Tube Feedings • 149
Assisting with Feedings • 151
Summing Up • 152
Real-Life Scenario • 153
Purpose of the Activity • 154
Handouts and Transparency Masters • 155

Module 5

Recreation and Activities 177

General Information/Overview • 178
Activities • 178
Cognitive Abilities Needed to Complete Tasks • 179
Making an Activity Successful • 182
Functional Evaluation • 183
Wandering • 185
Reasons for Wandering • 186
Elopement-Prevention Programs • 187
Management of Wandering • 188
Fall Prevention • 192

Choosing an Activity • 193
Summing Up • 197
Real-Life Scenario • 199
Purpose of the Activity • 200
Handouts and Transparency Masters • 201

Module 6 — Common Medical Problems 219

General Information/Overview • 220
The Normal Aging Process • 220
Normal Aging and Dementia • 226
Common Medical Problems • 227
Pressure Ulcers • 230
Dehydration • 231
Infections • 232
Medication • 232
Pain Management • 233
Pain Assessment • 235
Treatments for Pain • 236
Review of End-Stage Alzheimer's Disease • 237
End-of-Life (EOL) Care and Dementia • 237
Impending Death • 240
Summing Up • 241
Real-Life Scenario • 243
Purpose of the Activity • 244
Handouts and Transparency Masters • 245

Module 7 — Coping with Dementia 265

General Information and Overview • 266
Early in the Disease Process • 266
Changes in Role • 269
Responses to the Diagnosis of Dementia • 271
Emotions and Dementia • 273
Legal Issues • 274
Care Options • 275
Summing Up • 276
Real-Life Scenario • 277
Purpose of the Activity • 278
Handouts and Transparency Masters • 279

Module 8 — Caring for the Caregiver 291

General Information/Overview • 292
Burdens of Caregiving and Caregiver Burnout • 292
Informal Caregivers • 293
Formal Caregivers • 294
The Effects of Caregiver Burden • 295
Stress • 295
Conquering the Effects of Caregiver Burden and Burnout • 297
Techniques to Reduce Stress • 298

Healthy Living • 300
Reducing Risk Factors • 301
Stress and Elder Abuse • 302
Categories of Elder Abuse • 303
Types of Abuse • 304
Who Abuses • 307
Summing Up • 308
Real-Life Scenario • 309
Purpose of the Activity • 310
Handouts and Transparency Masters • 311

References **335**

Resources **337**

Answers to Pre- and Post-Tests **339**

Introduction

With the increase in life expectancy in the United States, society is faced with accompanying challenges in health care. The portion of the population over the age of 65 is growing rapidly and will reach an estimated 20% by 2030. With aging comes the risk of chronic and degenerative illnesses. Alzheimer's disease and related dementias are the eighth leading cause of death in the United States. "Dementia" is a general term or condition describing persons with brain impairment impacting their cognitive and memory functioning. Dementia usually occurs in the second half of life, primarily over the age of 65. When Dr. Alzheimer first met his patient in 1906, he was unaware of the role this affliction would play in the twenty-first century.

The role of health care is to support and enhance the quality of life of those affected with dementia. Training and education are essential to accomplish this goal. *Dementia Care Inservice Modules for Long-Term Care* is an all-inclusive set of inservices dedicated to the care of individuals with Alzheimer's disease and related dementia. Each of the eight, one-hour inservice modules is created to decrease preparation time for the presenter by including current research materials, a computer disc compatible with Microsoft PowerPoint®, transparency masters, pre- and post-tests, and handouts. Each module is concluded with summaries, real-life scenarios, and group activities to further the learning process. *Dementia Care Inservice Modules for Long-Term Care* prepares any member of the health care team for the daily ups and downs of dementia caregiving.

● RELATED PRODUCTS AVAILABLE FROM THOMSON DELMAR LEARNING:

- Kuhn Verity, *Providing Good Care to People with Dementia*, ISBN 140189951X
- Cobble Hill Health Center, *Speaking from Experience: Nursing Assistants Share Their Knowledge of Dementia Care*, ISBN 1401844146
- Pillemer, *Family Members Survival Guide: What Every Relative of a Nursing Home Resident Needs to Know*, ISBN 1401848206

ACKNOWLEDGMENTS

The authors and Thomson Delmar Learning wish to thank the following reviewers for their comments and suggestions on this manuscript:

Judy Billiman, RN
Corporate Education Services Manager
Five Star Quality Care
Newton, MA

Suzette Bos
Nursing Staff Development Coordinator
Austin Medical Center
Austin, MN

Deborah Drexler, Ms, RN, BC
Director of Clinic Nursing
Fond du Lac Regional Clinic
Fond du Lac, WI

Marie Moran, RN, BA
Staff Development
Loveland Good Samaritan Village
Loveland, CO

Janice Tolman, RN, BSPA
Director of Clinical Services
Mariner Health Care
Atlanta, GA

Patricia Trapp, RN, MAE
Staff Educator
Beaver Dam Community Hospital, Inc.
Columbus, WI

Effective Teaching Strategies

Effective teaching strategies should be incorporated into all training programs to promote learning and effectiveness. A successful inservice presentation is the combination of accurate research material and the ability to keep the audience attentive. Utilize the following strategies, with the enclosed modules, to enhance the delivery of the training session.

Be Enthusiastic

Use enthusiasm when presenting information. The audience needs to believe the presenter's excitement, to gain interest in the topic. Maintain eye contact with everyone in the audience by changing positions and direction when speaking. Use body language to emphasize critical points.

Use Humor

Make the presentation as entertaining as possible. Use humor to reduce anxiety and maintain the students' attention. There is no need to make a production of the event.

Take Risks

Embrace new teaching methods. Each audience is unique and may require a different approach to learning. Taking risks empowers the presenter to learn as well.

Incorporate Real-Life Examples

Whenever possible, incorporate real-life examples into the presentation. Often the lecture material is technical and dry; learners want to know why the topic is important to them.

Be Flexible

Flexibility is the characteristic of a good teacher. The group or audience often dictates the mood of the presentation. The instructional method may need to vary with group size or topic. During the presentation, observe the audience's reactions and demeanor. Adjust the teaching method to match the learner's needs.

Initiate Thought-Provoking Activities

Learning involves comparing new experiences with past experiences and gaining a new understanding. Initiate thought-provoking activities by posing questions, brainstorming, and testing to advance problem-solving skills.

Be Prepared

Be well prepared for the inservice. Research material should be thoroughly reviewed prior to class time. Answer questions honestly even if the answer is unknown. Do not give false information. Direct questioners to sources where the information can be found, such as organizations, books, and articles.

Get Feedback

Seek feedback from the audience to evaluate the quality of the lecture. Solicit remarks at the end of each presentation through evaluations or pre- and post-tests. Knowing the audience's perception of the inservice helps gauge strengths and weaknesses. During each session, observe the audience's non-verbal communication such as lack of eye contact or restlessness. Unite the audience by querying their understanding of the material. Alter the teaching strategy accordingly.

Reinforce Important Items

Strengthen the learning process by repeating key information. Reinforce the information with clear statements emphasizing what is important for the audience to remember. Utilizing the following statements in the discussion: "again we see," "as mentioned before," or "remember."

Summarize Key Points

At the end of any teaching session, summarize the important points. This reinforces the teaching-learning process and provides feedback on the progress made.

Tips for Using the PowerPoint Presentation

The use of visual aides during a presentation enhances the audience's experience. Combining what is heard with what is seen elevates the level of learning. Visual aids should enhance the presentation and not detract from the lecture material. The slides, poster boards, and other aids should display key elements of the inservice while the presenter expands the audience's knowledge. Remember to do the following:

- Expand on the information in the slides or provide complete handouts.
- Display one point on the screen at a time by masking the rest with a piece of paper. That way, the learner can concentrate on one idea at a time.
- Make sure the screen is large enough for the audience to read the information.
- Read from the screen the audience sees, not from the notes.
- When using an overhead projector, turn it off when it is not in use. The fan noise can be distracting.

Module 1
Understanding Dementia

Goal
To understand the causes of dementia and Alzheimer's disease.

Objectives
After completion of the presentation, students will be able to:

- Define the term *dementia*.
- List three types of dementia.
- Describe a diagnostic evaluation for Alzheimer's disease.
- Describe the process of diagnosing a client with Alzheimer's disease.
- Explain the phrase "probable Alzheimer's disease."
- Describe the seven stages of Alzheimer's disease.
- Describe the importance of observation, reporting, and the role of the nursing assistant.
- Describe how to report a change in a client's condition.

DEMENTIA FOR LONG-TERM CARE

Lecture Material for Slide 1-1

GENERAL INFORMATION/OVERVIEW

Dementia is a general term describing a person with a brain impairment impacting cognitive and memory functioning. The term *Alzheimer's disease* (*AD*) dates back to 1906, when Dr. Alois Alzheimer, a German physician practicing in Frankfurt-am-Main, Germany, presented a medical case. The case described a 51-year-old female with a five-year history of progressive mental deterioration, marked by irrational jealousy, increasing confusion, memory loss, and the inability to care for herself. With the introduction of a new staining technique, Dr. Alzheimer autopsied her brain and found disorganization of nerve cells in the part of the brain responsible for memory and reasoning. He documented the brain changes and published his findings in a medical journal in 1907. Similar findings were found in other patients who exhibited the same cognitive decline. A prominent German psychiatrist, Emil Kraepelin, suggested the new disease be named after Dr. Alzheimer.

- Dementia is a symptom of an illness, most commonly associated with Alzheimer's disease. In Latin *dementia* means irrationality. Dementia and Alzheimer's disease are not normally part of aging.

- Dementia symptoms include the loss of mental faculties relating to memory, personality, and behavior. Alzheimer's disease was once considered a psychiatric disorder, not a medical illness.

- Dementia usually occurs in the second half of life, primarily over the age of 65. It is estimated that one in 10 persons over the age of 65 has Alzheimer's disease and nearly one half of people over the age of 85 are afflicted with this disease.

- According to the U.S. Census Bureau, between the years 2000 and 2030, the number of people over the age of 65 will double; hence the number of people with AD will increase.

- The number of new cases of AD will peak in 2040 when the baby boomers reach the age of 65 and older.

- Presently, an estimated 4.5 million people have AD. Half of all nursing home residents suffer from Alzheimer's disease or other forms of dementia.

- If new treatments do not become available, by 2050, 13.2 million older Americans are expected to have AD (NIA 2004).

- The national cost to care for people with AD is about $100 billion per year. The cost of having a family member with AD is more than financial. The families suffer emotional and mental distress as well.

- The exact cause of AD is still not fully known. Most researchers agree the disease is caused by an array of factors.

Lecture Material for Slide 1-2

TYPES OF DEMENTIA

Dementia describes a group of symptoms reflecting abnormal brain function. Dementia is an impairment of a person's intellectual functioning. Symptoms include forgetting familiar people, ignoring basic safety, and failing to meet nutritional needs. Dementia usually impacts the activities of daily living. Dementia is not a normal part of aging and is not a disease in itself. The term *dementia* has replaced the once used diagnoses of senility and organic brain syndrome.

Symptoms of dementia include:
- Frequently repeating the same question.
- Getting lost driving to familiar places.
- Becoming very forgetful.
- Having difficulty with daily tasks.
- Changes in personality and frequent mood swings.
- Unable to follow simple commands.
- Overlooking safety hazards.
- Having poor personal hygiene.
- Being disoriented to people, places, and time.

Reversible Dementia

- Dementia is caused by many conditions. When the cause of the dementia is directly related to a treatable medical problem, the symptoms are reversible or will improve.
- Treatable conditions that can cause dementia include dehydration, elevated body temperature, infections, vitamin deficiency, and poor nutrition. Other possibilities are adverse reactions to medicines, thyroid deficiency, or a minor brain injury.
- Depression is common in the elderly population and can manifest memory loss, confusion, and other defects. Whenever a person with cognitive loss is depressed, an evaluation is needed to determine whether the depression causes the symptoms of dementia or dementia causes the depression.

Irreversible Dementia

Irreversible dementia is when the dementia is progressive and incurable. Multi-infarct dementia (MID) and Alzheimer's disease are the most common forms of irreversible dementia.

Multi-Infarct Dementia (MID)

- MID, or vascular dementia, is a result of a series of mini strokes or changes in the brain's blood supply. Narrowing or blockages of arterial blood to the brain is the usual cause.
- The onset is usually steplike in nature. The person "gets worse" after the stroke, rather than gradually changing as in Alzheimer's disease.
- The location of the stroke determines the seriousness of the problem and symptoms. If the symptoms appear slowly, it may be difficult to distinguish the signs from AD.

- The leading cause of MID is high blood pressure. Identifying and treating the cause of repeated strokes can prevent further damage.
- Unlike AD, multi-infarct dementia may show signs of improvement or a plateau of symptoms.
- A person may have both Alzheimer's disease and MID.

Alzheimer's Disease (AD)

- AD is the most common form of dementia and will be discussed at length during this lecture.
- AD is a progressive, degenerative disease, which affects the neurons of the brain causing them to die at an abnormally increased rate. This prevents the brain from working properly.
- In the beginning stages of AD, the remaining neurons can overcompensate for the neurons being lost. Research shows four out of five neurons can be destroyed before any symptoms are noticed.
- Once the symptoms begin to show, the disease is considered irreversible. Memory loss, changes in behavior, and language skills are commonly noted. Research suggests the disease is multifactored with environment and genetics.

Huntington's Disease

Huntington's disease is an inherited progressive disorder involving degeneration of nerve cells in the brain. The progressive loss of mental function includes abnormal body movements, dementia, and psychiatric problems.

Dementia with Lewy Bodies (Lewy Body Disease)

Lewy body disease is a neurodegenerative disorder causing dementia-like symptoms. The disorder is associated with abnormal structures called Lewy bodies. Lewy bodies have been found in the brain of Parkinson's and Alzheimer's clients and may be a variation of both diseases rather than a distinctive disorder.

Parkinson's Disease

Parkinson's disease also causes a slow progressive form of dementia usually noted in people over the age of 70. The dementia results from loss of nerve cells, which are needed to produce the neurotransmitters, dopamine, norepinephrine, or acetylcholine.

Frontal Lobe Dementia (Pick's Disease)

Frontal lobe dementia is characterized by gradual changes in personality, concentration, social interaction, motivation, and decision-making skills. In this type of dementia, memory is not affected in the early stages and may commonly be misdiagnosed as a psychiatric disorder. The main difference between frontal lobe dementia and Alzheimer's disease is the location of the initial damage of the brain. The frontal and temporal lobes of the brain are first affected with frontal lobe dementia. Damage occurring with Alzheimer's disease affects the temporal and parietal lobes first.

AIDS-Related Dementia

HIV infection of the brain occurs early after initial exposure to the virus, probably within the first few months, and remains clinically silent. The initial trigger that causes the emergence of AIDS dementia, in some patients, after years of silent brain infection is unknown. The development of certain neurovirulent HIV strains, due to mutation of the virus, may be a cause.

Mild Cognitive Impairment (MCI)

MCI is a condition characterized by mild recent memory loss, without dementia or significant impairment of other cognitive functions. The memory complaint is focused on short-term recall and abnormal memory for the chronological age. The overall cognitive functioning is normal. Eighty percent of people with MCI will develop AD within 10 years. Many experts suggest MCI is a precursor of AD rather than a distinct condition.

Lecture Material for Slide 1-3

● THE NORMAL HUMAN BRAIN

The human brain is the powerhouse of the human body. The perfected structure is responsible for sensory, motor, and intellectual functioning. The brain is also responsible for emotions, breathing, hunger, and digestion. When the brain is affected, so are all its functions.

- The human brain is a highly structured mass of nervous tissue. The brain weighs approximately three pounds and is made of billions of neurons (brain cells). These neurons work together in harmony through a series of intricate chemical signals to store, process, and retrieve information.
- The fragile mass is protected by a bony structure called the cranial cavity.

Cerebrum

- The cerebrum is the largest portion of the brain containing two symmetrical structures connected by a thick bundle of nerves called the corpus callosum. Each hemisphere is subdivided into four lobes. Each lobe is responsible for different activities and will be discussed in detail later in this module.
- The outer layer of neurons is called the cerebral cortex.
- All sensory information is received and processed in this area (sight, hearing, feeling, taste, smell). The cerebrum controls conscious thoughts, decision making, speech, communication, and other mental activities.
- The cerebrum also controls voluntary movements, such as getting up from a chair on demand.

Cerebellum

- The cerebellum is responsible for balance and coordination, by receiving information from the eyes, ears, and muscles regarding body position. Walking and spontaneously turning around are the result of a properly functioning cerebellum.
- Damage to the cerebellum may result in ataxia or problems with muscle coordination. This damage can interfere with a person's ability to walk, talk, eat, and perform other self-care tasks.

Brain Stem

- Neurological functions located in the brain stem include those necessary for survival (breathing, digestion, heart rate, blood pressure) and for arousal (being awake and alert).
- The spinal cord is connected to the brain by the brain stem.

Limbic System

- The limbic system controls muscle tone, emotions, and the storing of memories.
- It includes the hippocampus and parts of the cerebral cortex.
- Damage to the limbic system may also lead to alteration in smell, sexual behavior, and emotions.

Hippocampus

- Pronounced hip-o-KAM-pus, this portion of the brain is located in the cerebrum and is part of the limbic system.
- This portion of the brain is usually first to be affected by AD. Its function includes placing new memories into storage and allowing short-term memories to be converted into long-term memories.
- Damage to this area results in short-term memory loss, repetitive questioning, and confusion.

Hypothalamus

- The hypothalamus sits above the brain stem and is considered the control center of the brain.
- The hypothalamus produces hormones that regulate thirst, hunger, body temperature, sleep, and sexual behavior.
- Alternations in blood pressure, in the regulation of body temperature, in appetite control (satiety center), and in hydration are observed with damage to this area.

Amygdala

- Pronounced uh-MIG-duh-luh, this part of the limbic system is located in the temporal lobe. It functions to control the autonomic nervous

system (fight or flight response), as well as emotional and sexual behavior.
- Symptoms seen with damage include angry outburst, inappropriate sexual behavior, and fear.

Lecture Material for Slide 1-4

● NEURONS

Within the separate areas of the brain are approximately 140 billion specialized nerve cells, called neurons. The role of the neuron is to transmit a message from one neuron to another to complete a task. Their job is to generate electrical and chemical impulses, which relay information throughout the brain and nervous system.

- Each neuron has extensions called dendrites and axons, which help with the transmission of nerve impulses. An axon transmits messages to other neurons, while the dendrites receive messages from axons of neighboring neurons. A neuron may have several dendrites but only one axon.
- A synapse is a specialized area of communication between neurons. A neurotransmitter is a chemical that flows from the axon of one neuron to a receptor site on a dendrite of an adjacent neuron.
- The electrical impulse travels the length of the neuron, where the neurotransmitter is released. One class of neurotransmitters is acetylcholine (Ach), which is essential for cognitive function. Ach is the neurotransmitter for nerve and muscle cells.
- Neurons stay healthy by transporting nutrients found in circulating blood and converting them into energy.

Lecture Material for Slides 1-5 and 1-6

● NEURON CHANGES WITH AD

Alzheimer's disease causes damage to the brain by changing the structure of neurons and reducing the production of the neurotransmitter acetylcholine.

Slide 1-5

The Hallmark of AD

Dr. Alzheimer's discovery of beta-amyloid plaques and neurofibrillary tangles are known as the hallmarks of AD. Researchers are learning more about their formation, composition, and role in Alzheimer's disease.

Beta-Amyloid Plaques

- Beta-amyloid plaques are dense deposits of protein and cellular material that accumulate outside and around nerve cells (neurons).
- These plaques are formed from a protein found in neurons in the brain. The protein, amyloid precursor protein (APP), penetrates out through the nerve cell membrane. Certain enzymes cut the exposed

protein into fragments of protein, forming fibrils that cluster together. The fibrils, called beta-amyloid, begin to clump together, forming plaques. The plaques displace brain cells, eventually disrupting the work of neurons in the hippocampus and other areas of the cerebral cortex. Areas that are responsible for memories and other cognitive activities are being destroyed.

- In a healthy person, protein fragments would be reabsorbed and eliminated.
- Researchers are still unsure if the plaques cause AD or are a by-product of the disease.

Slide 1-6

Neurofibrillary Tangles

- Neurofibrillary tangles consist of clusters of insoluble twisted fibers found inside the neurons.
- Healthy neurons have an internal support structure partly made up of microtubules. The microtubules transport nutrients and other necessary elements through the brain cell for proper nutrition. A certain protein, tau, binds the microtubules together and forms a strong ladderlike infrastructure.
- With Alzheimer's disease, tau proteins loosen and tangle, causing the microtubules to disintegrate.
- As a result of the structure falling apart, the microtubules can no longer transport the nutrients needed to sustain the integrity of the neurons, and the cells die.

Lecture Material for Slide 1-7

● EFFECTS OF AD ON CEREBRAL FUNCTION

Neuron deaths begin slowly and continue for many years before any dementia symptoms are actually seen. Deterioration of function appears only after 30% of brain cell loss according to research. During the presymptomatic period, the remaining neurons are able to compensate for the brain cell death. As the disease devours the brain cells, the AD client is no longer able to process his or her surroundings. The client needs to use other functioning portions of the brain to complete tasks. Understanding the amount of brain function loss is necessary to determine what the client is able to process. The following reviews each lobe or section of the human brain and its specific functions.

Frontal Lobe

- The frontal lobe is located behind the forehead and significantly influences personality. This lobe is associated with the higher mental activities such as planning, judgment, and conceptualizing.
- Damage may be noted by alteration in self-control, emotion, intellect, memory, speech, and morality. The change in personality is extremely difficult for family members.

- This lobe of the brain is also responsible for levels of concentration, attention span, safety, and proper judgment. AD impairs people's judgment, causing them to become easily distracted and lessening their initiative.

Audience Interaction for Slide 1-7

How can the caregiver best help a client with frontal lobe defects?

- Give step-by-step directions for completing a task. Use cues or prompts to start an activity. Most activities of daily living require many decisions. When dressing, decide what is weather-appropriate, what matches, and so on. Lay out the outfit for the client to wear. Make sure the clothes are in the correct order of application. Keep it simple.
- Reduce safety hazards in the environment.
- Reduce distractions.

Parietal Lobe

- The parietal lobe, also referred to as the association area, is located above the ears and interprets pain sensation, pressure, temperature, and touch.
- Damage to this area can cause visuospacial disturbances or problems with visual perception (eg, clients may have difficulty finding their way around new or even familiar places).
- Impairment of the parietal lobe may also disrupt a client's ability to understand spoken and/or written language.
- The parietal lobes contain the primary sensory cortex, which controls sensation such as touch and pressure. The association area controls fine sensation, including judgment of texture, weight, size, and shape. Clients may be hunched over because of their loss of spatial dimension.

Audience Interaction for Slide 1-7

How can the caregiver best help a client with parietal lobe defects?

- Assist the client by using cues and gestures, and body language.
- Use a prompt to explain the purpose of an object. Mimic the actions of brushing teeth when holding a toothbrush.

Temporal Lobe

- There are two temporal lobes, located at ear level, one on each side of the brain.
- The functions of the temporal lobes include hearing, understanding sounds, emotions, memory, and the ability to draw. These areas allow a person to distinguish one smell from another and one sound from another. The temporal lobes assist in sorting new information and are believed to be responsible for short-term memory.
- The client with damage to the temporal lobe will have aphasia, or impaired language. If cell death occurs to the right lobe, disruptions in memories of pictures and faces occurs (visual memory). If the damage takes place in the left side, memory loss for words and names emerges (verbal memory).

Audience Interaction for Slide 1-7

How can the caregiver best help a client with temporal lobe defects?
- During the early stages of the disease, try to fill in the missing words for the client. The client may benefit from books on tape to ease the burden of reading.
- As the disease worsens, the use of gestures, body language, and physical prompts helps.

Occipital Lobe

- The occipital lobe is located at the back of the head and processes visual information. It also contains areas that help in the visual recognition of shapes and colors.
- The information received from the eyes referencing the body's orientation, position, and movement is interpreted in this area.
- Damage to this lobe can cause visual deficits. Defects lead to a loss of depth perception peripheral vision, as well as difficulty processing rapid movements.

Audience Interaction for Slide 1-7

How can the caregiver best help a client with occipital lobe defects?
- With visual disturbance, it is recommended to approach the client from the front.
- Use eye contact.
- Use slow movements.
- Avoid floor and wall designs that could be misinterpreted. For example, a black and white tile floor could appear to the AD client as many holes in the floor.

Lecture Material for Handout 1-2

Review Handout 1-2 with the audience. The information reinforces the content previously discussed or can act as a review session for future lectures.

AD Analogy

If we use an orchestra as an analogy for AD, we can visualize the affects of brain cell death. If one violinist misses a note, the music changes only slightly and only to those with an educated ear. As more musicians miss notes, the music becomes distorted for only a moment at a time. When the whole string section is off-key, the horn section and eventually all parts of the orchestra become affected; the music becomes noise. The damaged brain can no longer conceptualize a thought, feeling, or action.

Lecture Material for Slide 1-8

● FACTORS INCREASING THE RISK FOR AD

Research has led to numerous theories about the underlying cause of Alzheimer's disease. Studies have not been able to determine if there is only one cause. The research has shown there may be multiple factors contributing to the development of AD, including environmental toxins, genetics, and viruses. Identifying and reducing risk factors will lead to new treatments and prevention strategies.

Aging

- Many studies have concluded the greatest risk for developing AD is age. The number of people diagnosed with AD doubles every year past the age of 65. The average age of diagnosis is 80.
- Some of the neurons in a healthy person shrink and work less efficiently; some brain cell death is a normal part of aging. However, research shows that the neurons responsible for learning do not die in a healthy aging person. Only when the numbers of unhealthy and dead neurons outnumber the healthy neurons can the memory loss no longer be considered a normal part of aging.
- AD is not commonly seen in middle-aged people, and less frequently seen in persons in their thirties. Early-onset Alzheimer's is classified when the person is 65 years of age or younger. The younger the age of the client at diagnosis, the more rapid the progression. However, early onset does not mean the person is in the first stage of the disease. Many times a person of such an age is misdiagnosed because of their overall health. Health care professionals, as well as friends and family, attribute the cognitive decline to stress, depression, or other psychiatric illness.

Heredity and Genetics

A family history of AD, especially a first-degree blood relative (parent or sibling), increases the risk of developing the disease, making it one and a half to two times greater than the risk for those without a family history. How the disease is passed on through unidentified genetic mutations or why it may affect only one family member is not yet understood.

Familial

Familial Alzheimer's, an inherited form of the disease, accounts for less than 10% of AD cases. This early-onset form of the disease usually strikes during middle age. The genetic mutation is located on one of three chromosomes (1, 14, or 21). Alzheimer's disease develops if the mutation is present. Genetic testing for this form of AD is reliable. An individual has a 50% chance of developing the disease if one parent has been diagnosed.

Sporadic

The more common form of the disease, late-onset, does not have a clear genetic link. Researchers know that individuals born with gene ApoE4 are at greater risk for developing the disease than those with gene ApoE2. The more common gene, ApoE3, has no effect on the likelihood of developing the disease. Since all gene types still may develop the disease, testing is not recommended. Scientists are studying other genetic and environmental factors, which may help with unraveling the mystery of the disease.

Health History

A health history includes detailed information regarding past and present illnesses of the client and extended family members.

Cardiovascular Factors

Researchers have investigated the influence of hypertension (HTN) and hypercholesterolemia (elevated blood cholesterol levels) on the development of AD. Each is linked to the cause of cardiovascular disease, which is directly related to strokes. People with HTN or high blood levels of cholesterol are twice as likely of developing AD. Those with both risk factors are four times more likely to develop dementia.

History of Head Trauma

Studies have reported suffering a head injury with a loss of consciousness increases the risk of developing AD later in life.

Down Syndrome

Another genetic link to developing AD is Down syndrome, a chromosomal defect located on chromosome 21 resulting in mental retardation. On autopsy, all middle-aged persons with the syndrome have defects in the brain tissue consistent with AD; not all persons exhibit symptoms.

Lecture Material for Slides 1-9 and 1-10

Slide 1-9

SIGNS AND SYMPTOMS OF DEMENTIA

Symptoms of AD begin slowly. The person may forget a familiar place, a person's name, or recent events. The phrases "senior moment" or "I keep forgetting things; I must be getting Alzheimer's" have become common expressions. The act of forgetting a single incident is not a sign of dementia. Forgetting where the keys are placed is a common occurrence and not a reason for concern. AD causes the person not to know the purpose of the keys or the ability to trace back to where the keys were last seen.

- The symptoms initially are perceived more as a nuisance than a concern. Many times, the family is unaware of the mild impairment. The client often covers up the memory loss.

- People with AD do not regress to their childhood. The brain no longer has the capacity to make decisions or complete tasks; so the thought process or developmental age mimics that of a child.

- As the disease progresses, all higher brain functions diminish. Any task requiring executive functioning (the ability to follow a series of steps) and/or abstract thinking (the ability to think in terms of ideas) exemplifies the defect. For example, a person will have difficulty setting the table for a meal, planning a vacation, or socializing.

- When the disease advances, changes in mood and behavior are commonly seen. Research suggests the cause may be linked to neuron damage in the communication and limbic system.

Warning Signs

The Alzheimer's Association has developed a checklist of warning signs for AD. It describes common symptoms seen in the early stages. If symptoms persist or worsen, further evaluation is suggested. A single event is not a precursor of dementia.

Increasing and Continuing Forgetfulness
- Forgetting current events, conversations, and names of objects.
- Repeating the same sentence or thought.

Difficulty Performing Familiar Tasks
- Difficulty using a toaster
- Problems brushing teeth
- Unable to dial a common phone number

Problems with Language
- Difficulty with word searching
- Inability to express thoughts
- Difficulties in reading and writing.

Poor Judgment
- Buying unnecessary and expensive items from telemarketers
- Giving away large sums of money for no apparent reason
- Wearing clothing inappropriate for the weather (too many clothes in the summer and not enough clothes in the winter)

Problems with Abstract Thinking
- Inability to reconcile a checkbook
- Difficulty planning a menu for dinner

Misplacing Items
- Inappropriate placing of items (reading glasses in the freezer, food in the clothes closet)
- Difficulty identifying the item itself

Mood/Personality and Behavior Changes
- Mood swings without provocation
- Episodes of aggression with outbursts
- Feelings of depression and distrust

Loss in Initiative
- Loss of interest in hobbies
- Loss of motivation
- Passive behavior
- Sleeping more than usual

Lecture Material for Slide 1-11

⬤ DIAGNOSTIC EVALUATION

Anyone with memory problems needs to have a comprehensive diagnostic evaluation. Evaluation is the only way to determine the cause of the impairments. AD is not the only possible cause for amnesia-type memory impairment. Symptoms may originate from normal aging (age-related cognitive decline) or mild cognitive impairment.

- A physician can complete an informal interview if there is concern over cognitive loss. The client is interviewed with a reliable informant present to help with clinical history and general information. Impaired memory may be seen in the way a person responds to simple questions, in word searching, and in direct complaints. For example, the client is unable to recall recent events, tells of forgetting a meal on the stove when cooking, misplaces keys, wallet, or other items. Observations are made on how the client reacts when a question is asked. Does he or she turn and look at the family member/caregiver to provide the answer. The client may lack insight and require verification. Once the cognitive decline is evident, a more formal assessment is needed.

- A diagnostic evaluation also provides reassurance for aging individuals who are not symptomatic but who are concerned about possible memory decline in the future. For these individuals, a diagnostic evaluation provides a baseline for future assessments.

- The diagnostic evaluation has a multitude of components, including a detailed history of the onset and progression of symptoms. Family members are present to verify the accuracy of information. The evaluation reviews all medical history, medications, mental health, and laboratory and neurological testing.

A Complete Physical Exam

- A complete history and physical examination is performed to determine if the dementia is the result of an underlying illness. Conditions of the thyroid, hypertension, heart arrhythmia, electrolyte imbalances, and vitamin B_{12} deficiency are investigated.

- Neuroimaging plays an important role in excluding alternative causes of dementia. Magnetic resonance imaging (MRI) or a computed tomography (CT) scan shows images of the brain, ruling out stroke, brain tumors, or hydrocephalus. Positron emission tomography (PET) and single photon emission computer tomography (SPECT) can increase the ability to predict cognitive decline, thus offering early diagnosis and treatment.

Psychiatric Evaluation

Psychiatric evaluation assesses the client for cognitive ability; evaluates memory, concentration, and orientation. It examines how the person functions, looking at behavior and mood in everyday situations.

Psychometric Testing

- Psychometric testing determines whether the brain is functioning properly. These tests objectively measure cognitive function, including accuracy, speed, and the quality of the thought process. Recent and past memory, concentration, language, and problem-solving skills are part of the cognitive function. Such patterns provide useful information and assist the health care professional in providing treatment strategies for the client.

- The most commonly used assessment scale to establish the presence of dementia is the Mini-Mental State Examination (MMSE), developed by Marshal F. Folstein. The test asks questions related to orientation to time and place, calculations, recall, language, attention, following commands, and spatial perception. Each task is given a number value with a maximum score of 30 points. Scores less than 24 suggest dementia. The test scores must be adjusted for clients with mild dementia, low education level, or impaired vision.

Sample questions include:
- What season is it?
- Spell "world" backward.
- Repeat the phrase "No ifs ands or buts."
- Redraw an image from this picture.

Lecture Material for Slide 1-12

● DIAGNOSING ALZHEIMER'S DISEASE

Alzheimer's disease is a clinical diagnosis with no definitive test to confirm its presence. The diagnosis is ascertained from ruling out other disorders and illnesses.

Clinical Diagnosis of AD

In 1984, a criteria for the clinical diagnosis of AD was developed by the National Institute of Neurological and Communicative Disorders and Stroke and the Alzheimer's Disease and Related Disorders Association (now known as the Alzheimer's Association.). The criteria have three levels of diagnostic certainty: possible, probable, and definitive.

Possible AD

A diagnosis of possible AD is made when the symptoms are not typical of AD, but other disorders have been ruled out. Possible AD may be diagnosed if the client has an additional underlying illness that exhibits symptoms of dementia.

Probable AD

When the diagnostic evaluation excludes other causes of cognitive decline, and a historical pattern of functional and behavioral disturbances is noted, the diagnosis is probable AD. No histological confirmation is obtained. Specialized physicians who follow established guidelines can diagnose probable AD with 85% to 95% accuracy. (ADEAR)

Definite AD

Diagnosis of this class is made when histological confirmation is made. Brain tissue is examined and viewed for tangles and plaques. A biopsy can be obtained from a living source but this is rare; most occur at time of autopsy. The clinical diagnosis of AD is accurate, with autopsy studies confirming diagnoses in more than 80% of the cases.

Disclosing the Diagnosis

- Commonly, family members want to shield their loved ones from the diagnosis of AD.
- The physician or family may avoid the term "Alzheimer's disease" or not mention the findings at all. Disclosing the diagnosis enables people with the disease to participate in their health care decisions. In addition, receiving the diagnosis may eliminate the need to cover up their confusion. Many clients do not grasp the full implications of the disease, possibly the only merciful part of the illness. Some people are relieved by the diagnoses and less embarrassed by their behavior and need for help.
- Early diagnosis plays an important role in the treatment of AD even though no cure or treatment for halting the disease is available. Theorists believe introducing medications at the first sign of impairment may delay the onset and progression of symptoms long enough for clients to live most of their natural lives unaffected. At the very least, early diagnosis allows clients and families to plan together for symptom management and care options, as well as to formulate treatment strategies.

STAGE OF AD

The Alzheimer's Association bases its staging protocol on the Global Deterioration Scale (GDS), developed by Dr. Barry Reisberg. This staging scale denotes the characteristics of AD symptom progression. The stages range from one to seven. A simplified scale refers to three stages: early, moderate, and late-stage AD. Both scales will be reviewed.

Symptoms of Alzheimer's disease begin slowly and become steadily worse. The stages are based on patterns of behaviors.

- As the disease progresses, symptoms range from mild forgetfulness to serious impairments in thinking, judgment, and the ability to perform daily activities.
- The disease progresses differently for each individual. Some people may or may not experience all the symptoms. Eventually, all clients need total care.
- During the disease the client has changes in cognition, affect, and physical condition.
- The average life expectancy postdiagnosis is eight years but can range from three to 20 years.

How to Use Staging

Reisberg's Brief Cognitive Rating Scale (BCRS) and Functional Assessment Staging (FAST) provide scores based on interview criteria measuring concentration, recent and past memory, orientation, and functioning/self-care. This score, divided by five, reflects a stage on the GDS. These specific assessment tools help health care professionals and caregivers determine treatments and special needs for the client.

The Global Deterioration Scale for Assessment of Primary Degenerative Dementia

Stage 1: Normal adult

- No cognitive decline
- No complaints of memory loss and no deficits assessed during a clinical interview

Stage 2: Very mild cognitive decline

- Age-associated memory impairment.
- Normal older adult with complaints of forgetfulness, most commonly forgetting names of people and where they placed objects, with awareness of the memory deficits.
- No difficulties with employment or social events; during a clinical interview, no memory deficit noted.

Stage 3: Mild cognitive impairment

- At this stage, mild cognitive decline is noted. The deficits are manifested in more than one area. The client starts to get lost when traveling. Work-related performance begins to decline. Written material is not retained after reading. Remembering new people and places is difficult. The client may lose or misplace items of value.
- During clinical testing the client appears to have difficulty concentrating. The client starts to deny incidences of cognitive decline. Mild to moderate anxiety is usually present.

Slide 1-15 | *Stage 4: Moderate cognitive decline*

- This is the mild or early stage of AD (early stage using the simplified scale).
- Moderate cognitive loss is evident during this stage.
- Symptoms include decreased knowledge of current events. The client may forget personal history. There is a noted decline in the ability to handle finances, travel, and other complex tasks.
- The client may show no decline in orientation to time and person, recognition of familiar persons, or traveling to customary locations.
- The client withdraws from challenging situations and uses denial as a defense mechanism. Flattening of affect begins during this stage.

Slide 1-16 | *Stage 5: Moderately severe cognitive decline*

- The client shows moderate to midstage dementia.
- During this stage the client appears to be normal. No assistance with feeding or personal care is needed. Language, speech, and social interactions are maintained. The person loses their train of thought, frequently experiencing delusions, suspiciousness, and anxiety.
- Moderately severe cognitive decline is noted at this stage. The client needs some form of assistance for survival; his or her understanding of reality is based on misperceptions.
- Clients are unable to name the relevant aspects of their lives, such as addresses, telephone numbers, and names of their grandchildren or of their alma mater.
- Clients are aware of their own names, their spouses and children's names, and the major facts about their lives and those closest to them. The disorientation is with time or place.

Slide 1-17 | *Stage 6: Severe cognitive decline*

- Clients exhibit moderately severe dementia (moderate stage using the simplified scale).
- Severe cognitive decline is documented. Clients are no longer oriented to time and place.
- They can recall their own names and can distinguish between familiar and unfamiliar people. They have some memories of the past but are unable to recall recent events. They may have difficulty counting backward from 10. Cognitive abulla (loss of initiative because the person is unable to maintain a thought process long enough to complete a task) is present.
- The client requires assistance with activities of daily living (ADL) and may experience incontinence.
- Personality and emotional changes occur. Behavioral problems include delusions, obsessive symptoms, anxiety, and depression. The client may continually repeat simple activities such as cleaning the same area.

Slide 1-18 | *Stage 7: Very severe cognitive decline*

- Clients exhibit late dementia/severe dementia (late stage using the simplified scale).
- This stage is depicted by severe cognitive decline. The client requires total care for all activities of daily living (ADL).
- Communication is limited to grunting. Basic psychomotor skills are lost. The client is unable to walk and sit up without assistance. By the end of this stage, the client has little to no head control.
- Like an infant, the client seeks immediate sensory gratification and can easily be overstimulated. Unfamiliar persons may experience resistance when providing personal care. The client accepts some interaction but initiates none.
- The brain no longer has the capacity to tell the mind to think, the soul to feel, or the body to move.
- In the late stages, the clients die from secondary illness and comorbid conditions, not from Alzheimer's disease.

Lecture Material for Slide 1-19

● TREATMENTS FOR AD

Treatment modalities for Alzheimer's disease have changed significantly with the new understanding of the disease process. Medical care of the symptoms has changed from palliative in nature to management of the disease. With early diagnosing, medications can begin to work before cognitive defects advance, ultimately prolonging the person's quality of life. The goal of Alzheimer's research is to develop disease-modifying medications leading to a cure.

Maintenance of Function

- During any stage of the disease, maximizing and maintaining both cognitive and functional abilities are crucial to maintaining quality of life. Utilizing medications to improve symptoms and slowing the progression of the disease impact the client's ability to carry out ADLs.
- Family support provides a layer of care that cannot be furnished by a facility. Information provided by families enables health care providers to formulate client-centered care. Incorporating the client's likes and dislikes into the care plan helps simulate their pre-illness persona. Each component of the treatment plan assists the client in adapting to the changing world.

Improving Symptoms

Utilizing drug therapy in the treatment of AD is aimed at improving memory and quality of life. The choice of medications can be based on side effects, dosing schedules, ease of use, individual response to a particular medication, or other factors.

Cholinesterase Inhibitors (ChEIs)

- Cholinesterase inhibitors work by delaying the breakdown of the neurotransmitter, acetylcholine. Acetylcholine helps communication between the nerve cells. AD causes a decreased level of this neurotransmitter. In the presence of ChEIs, more of the neurotransmitter is available to transmit messages.
- Cholinesterase inhibitors may delay cognitive decline for clients with mild to moderate AD. Studies have shown these drugs improve memory and the general ability to function. For example, clients may be able to remember friends' names and be able to dress themselves with less difficulty. ChEIs do not stop or reverse the destruction of brain cells, nor is the drug able to decrease the loss of acetylcholine.
- Cholinesterase inhibitors do not help everyone with Alzheimer's disease. As the disease progresses, the medication usually stops working.
- Cholinesterase inhibitors include Aricept® (donepezil hydrochloride), Razadyne® ERl® (galantamine hydrobromide), and Exelon® (rivastigmine tartrate).

Namenda® Memantine HCL

- The first Alzheimer's drug of this type approved in the United States, memantine is classified as a N-methyl-D-aspartate (NMDA) receptor antagonist. It is called a glutaminergic agent.
- The medication helps improve cognition by shielding the effects of excessive amounts of the neurotransmitter glutamate. The overexposure appears to be a major factor in cell injury and the death of brain cells in people with AD.
- The drug is found to be effective in moderate to severe forms of AD. It can assist the client and caregiver by prolonging the client's ability to carry out ADLs for a few extra months.

Behavioral Management

- Behavioral symptoms can be more burdensome than the amnesiac symptoms. Symptoms of agitation, anxiety, and irritability are common among all clients with AD, including those with mild dementia.
- The use of medications for behavioral symptoms are individualized for the client and family needs. The safety of the client, side effects of medications, and family support are all considerations when prescribing medications. Medications should target the specific behavior, not just general aggressive or agitated behaviors. Nondrug interventions should be the first line of defense.
- Psychotropic drugs are used for behavioral problems. These medications can reduce sleeplessness, depression, wandering, anxiety, and agitation.

Family Support

- Interviewing family members is the only way to learn about the client's background. By the time a client is placed in a facility, his or her cognitive function is diminished. Knowing a person's life story and traditions enhance all aspects of Alzheimer's care. Addressing the real person inside the shell of a dementia client can make the difference between a combative client and one who is a joy to be around.
- Communication is improved when the family can provide verbal cues for the client. Clients become less frustrated when their needs are met and understood.
- The client is comforted by conversations of interest. For example, if the client was an airline pilot, the caregiver can distract him or her with questions about planes when he or she becomes agitated. Reducing behavioral disturbances without medications is encouraged.

Slowing the Progression of AD

Medications aimed at slowing the disease progression hold the key to controlling this life-altering disease. Current clinical trials are testing compounds to help develop new treatment options. Studies include researching the affects of nonsteroidal anti-inflammatory drugs (NSAIDs), antioxidants, and vitamin E, as well as the use of ginkgo biloba, selegiline, and cholesterol-lowering drugs (statins). Research also includes medications to prevent the formation of beta-amyloid plaques and nerve growth factor to maintain healthy neurons.

Prevention of AD

- According to ongoing research, preventing AD is now thought to be an achievable goal. Even the Alzheimer's Association believes we can improve brain health.
- A healthy body and mind could be the first defense against AD. Eating a healthy diet, along with maintaining normal blood pressure, cholesterol levels, blood sugar, and body weight, may reduce the risk of AD.
- Adding an exercise regimen for the body and brain may also be beneficial. Studies have suggested that increasing the amount of leisure activity in daily life can increase and maintain cognitive function. This can be achieved by incorporating activities such as dance, exercise, reading, and crossword puzzles into daily routines.

● OBSERVATION AND REPORTING

Lecture Material for Slide 1-20

Various forms of information can be obtained by observing a client. The way clients interact with their environment provides information on their physical and mental capacity. Taking a virtual snapshot photo of the client at the initial meeting allows for continued comparison of the client's progress. Reporting changes in the client's condition to the supervisor can prevent complications, hospitalization, and even death. Stress the importance of reporting all the information to the supervisor, such as the amount of restlessness, outbursts, and emotional responses. Even subtle changes should not be overlooked; they can be cues for potential problems. The AD client does not have the cognitive ability to report problems.

Audience Interaction for Slide 1-20

Ask the audience to name the five senses and explain how each is used in observing a client with dementia.

The five senses are:

1. touch
2. sight
3. smell
4. hearing
5. taste

The Five Senses

- Using each of the five senses enables the caregiver to determine the client's level of functioning.
- Each sense can contribute information on how the client interacts with his or her environment. By detecting the smallest changes, the caregiver provides better care for the client.

Touch

- The sense of touch can provide the caregiver with important understanding of the client's need for personal space. The client's acceptance of an unfamiliar person is important to know when caring for those with Alzheimer's.
- A client can be reassured with touch. The caregiver can determine if such actions console a client or create more agitation.
- The physical attributes of skin are also assessable with touch: temperature, moisture, or pain. The client may be unable to express the simplest of needs.

Sight

- Vision is the easiest sense to use, but not always the easiest to explain. The overall appearance of the client should be noted.
- Take note on how the client interacts with the surroundings. If the client is still dressing himself or herself, are the clothing items donned properly? Is the apparel appropriate for the climate or season?

Smell

- The odor of a client can reflect his or her ability to complete personal hygiene or indicate incontinence.

- Infections or illnesses can also cause identifying odors. Diabetics can have a sweet smelling urine or acetone-smelling breath. Infections such as pseudomonas have a foul smell.

Hearing

- The physical assessment of breathing patterns; abnormal breath sounds such as wheezing or Cheyne-Stokes breathing (abnormal noisy breathing with periods of no breathing); and shortness of breath are detected using hearing.
- Listen to the client's fears or wants. Communication skills are maintained in the early stages of the disease. Clients lose their train of thought; so paying attention can be vital to understanding their needs.
- Observing how clients answer questions can give a sense of their cognitive ability and interactive skills. Dementia causes delusions, suspiciousness, and anxiety. Always determine the client's level of orientation to person, place, and time in order to provide a safe environment.

Taste

- Utilizing the client's sense of taste can help develop a nutritious diet. Dietary needs are a concern with the aging population and are compounded by the dementia.
- Observing food preferences can help with developing a nutritious meal plan. The Alzheimer's clients cannot always verbalize their wants. By watching their habits, the caregiver achieves a better understanding of their likes and dislikes.
- Remember clients may avoid certain foods on their plate, not because they do not like them, but because the food may appear unfamiliar.

Lecture Material for Slide 1-21

HOW TO REPORT CHANGES

Information relayed to the supervisor must be as accurate as possible. Make sure it is consistent with the actual findings. Describe what actually happened objectively, rather than giving a personal account of the situation. For example, "the client threw a dish at her husband" is more factual than "the client is fighting with her husband."

Objective Reporting

Objective reporting is the most accurate method of reporting; it is reporting exactly what is observed. The description is based on factual observations such as:

- "The sore on her leg is the size of a quarter."
- "Mrs. Smith is complaining of pain in her chest area."
- "My client is having shortness of breath; she cannot speak more than two-word sentences."

Subjective Reporting

Subjective reporting is the reporting of an opinion. The description is neither measurable nor comparable to other descriptions. Examples are:

- "The sore on her leg is big."
- "I think Mrs. Smith is having a heart attack."
- "My client cannot breathe."

Intuitions

- Gut feelings or intuitions have been an important source of reporting. The caregiver spends a lot of time with the client and often observes changes without being able to support them with objective (concrete) observations. Make the supervisor aware that this is a personal opinion or feeling when reporting this type information.

- During the disease process, the client with AD develops functional loss in communication, as well as changes in affect and physical condition. These changes occur at different times and to different degrees. Reporting the change in condition is what is important, not the use of technical jargon. Just stating to the supervisor, "I don't know what it is but Mr. Brown is not himself" is an appropriate comment. The supervisor may ask additional questions to better understand the problem, but the duty to report is met. Observation and reporting enables the health care team to provide the best treatment plan for the client.

Insert agency's policy here for reporting changes in client's condition.

SUMMING UP

Dementia is impairment in the intellectual functioning of a person caused by changes in the brain. Dementia is not a normal part of aging. Symptoms include the loss of mental faculties related to memory, personality, and behavior. As the number of brain cell deaths increase, the client's symptoms worsen. The impairments disrupt a person's ability to carry out normal activities of daily life. The most common cause of dementia is Alzheimer's disease, but it can be caused by other disorders.

Throughout this module emphasis has been placed on the functions of the brain and how the disease process alters a person's mind and abilities. Reporting all observations of the client's progress is one of the most important aspects of dementia care. Understanding how the brain is mutated can help caregivers assist with a client's weakness while promoting his or her strengths. With proper diagnosis and treatment options throughout the stages of AD, the client's care should remain individualized focusing on the person within.

Instructor's Version with Answers for Handout 1-3

● REAL-LIFE SCENARIO

A Day in the Life of Pat

Pat is a 72 year-old retired schoolteacher who lives alone. Pat is having increasing trouble completing the routine of grocery shopping. Pat complains to the store manager about the frequent changes in food placement and even accuses him of hiding the bathroom tissue. The store clerk helps Pat count the money needed to pay for the items. On one occasion, Pat wandered for over one hour in the parking lot looking for the car. When Pat's daughter arrived at the home she found the entire guest room filled with bathroom tissue and no food in the pantry. When confronted, Pat becomes angry and is unable to verbalize any thoughts.

1. List the possible warning signs for Alzheimer's disease, which Pat may be experiencing.
   - *Difficulty performing familiar tasks (grocery shopping).*
   - *Increasing and continuing forgetfulness (locating items in the grocery store and purchasing the same items).*
   - *Poor judgment (no food in the home).*
   - *Problems with abstract thinking (difficulty counting money).*
   - *Mood, personality, and behavior changes (accusing the store manager of hiding items).*
   - *Problems with language (unable to express thoughts when confronted).*

2. Pat's daughter contacted the primary physician for a diagnostic evaluation. What does a diagnostic evaluation include?

   A diagnostic evaluation for memory problems includes a complete physical exam, psychiatric evaluation, and psychometric testing.

3. According to the Global Deterioration Scale (GDS), what stage of Alzheimer's is Pat experiencing?

   According to GDS, Pat is in stage 5, moderately severe cognitive decline. The client appears to be normal and no assistance is needed with feeding or personal care. The person frequently experiences suspiciousness and anxiety. Some form of assistance is needed for survival.

GROUP ACTIVITY

● PURPOSE OF THE ACTIVITY

The purpose of this activity is to reinforce knowledge of the brain's anatomy and functions. The following activities can be completed as a class, small groups, or individually.

Option 1

Using Handout 1-2, have the students provide examples of the limitations a client with dementia may experience with damage in the following areas: cerebellum, brain stem, limbic system, hippocampus, hypothalamus, and amygdala.

Option 2

For the following behaviors, commonly observed with dementia clients, have the students determine where in the brain damage has occurred.

- Client is unable to dress himself.
- The client is agitated.
- The client loses her belongings.
- The client is unable to find the bathroom.
- The client has an angry outburst.
- The client uses the wrong words when speaking.
- The client has inappropriate sexual behavior.
- The client trips when walking.
- The client does not know what to do with a fork.

Name _____ Date _____

Program/Course _____ Instructor's Name _____

Understanding Dementia Pre- and Post-Test

1. The term dementia is a term used to describe:
   a. An individual with brain impairment impacting cognitive and memory functioning.
   b. An individual with below-normal intellectual function caused at birth.
   c. Intracranial hemorrhage.
   d. An individual with a brain tumor.

2. The most common cause of dementia is:
   a. Multi-infarct dementia.
   b. Parkinson's disease.
   c. Alzheimer's disease.
   d. Huntington's disease.

3. Brain cells are also called:
   a. Neons.
   b. Neurons.
   c. Klingons.
   d. Plaques.

4. A neurotransmitter is:
   a. An inflammation of a nerve or nerves.
   b. A chemical that transmits messages from one neuron to another to complete a task.
   c. A physician specializing in surgery of the nervous system.
   d. A toxin that attacks nerve tissue.

5. What are the hallmarks of Alzheimer's disease?
   a. Beta-amyloid plaques and neurofibrillary tangles
   b. Tangles
   c. Plaques
   d. Neuromyelitis and pleurisy

(continued)

Handout **1-1**

Understanding Dementia Pre- and Post-Test (Continued)

6. Name the sections of the cerebral cortex in the brain.
   a. Hypothalamus, brain stem, cerebellum, cortex
   b. Hypothalamus, thalamus, cerebral cortex
   c. Frontal lobe, temporal lobe, parietal lobe, occipital lobe
   d. Frontal lobe, parietal lobe, occipital lobe

7. Name two risk factors of Alzheimer's disease.
   a. Age and heredity
   b. Parkinson's disease and age
   c. Hypertension and AIDS
   d. Strokes and dementia

8. A common behavioral symptom observed with Alzheimer's disease is:
   a. Agitation.
   b. Ataxia.
   c. Vertigo.
   d. Numbness.

9. A diagnostic evaluation of Alzheimer's disease includes:
   a. CT scan and/or PET scan.
   b. A history and physical exam, psychiatric evaluation, and psychometric testing.
   c. An interview with family and/or caregivers.
   d. All of the above.

10. List three warning signs of dementia defined by the Alzheimer's Association.
    1. _____
    2. _____
    3. _____

Handout **1-1**

Cerebral Functions, Related Impairments, and Interventions

Areas of the brain	Functions	Impairment with dementia	Interventions
Frontal	• Judgment • Impulse control • Attention span • Organization • Problem solving • Empathy	• Lack of judgment • Impulsiveness • Easily distracted • Disorganization • Notable errors	• Give step-by-step directions. • Use cues to start a task. • Maintain safety. • Reduce distractions.
Temporal (left and right)	• Hearing/listening • Reading • Short-term memory • Recognition of objects • Anger control • Identification of objects by name • Visual memory • Verbal memory	• Aphasia • Reading problems • Short-term memory loss • Limited impulse control • Disruptions in memories for pictures and faces (right side) • Memory loss for words and names (left side)	• Assist the client with word searching. • Use gestures and body language. • Use physical prompts.
Parietal	• Sensations of touch, pressure, texture, and weight • Recognition of shape and size • Spatial recognition • Identifying the purpose of objects	• Inability to identify an object by touch, texture, weight, or size • Impaired sense of position • Inability to identify an object's purpose	• Use cueing. • Use body language to demonstrate. • Use prompts to show an item's purpose.
Occipital	• Sight • Visual interpretations • Depth perception • Self-orientation and positioning	• Visual problems • Visual illusions and hallucinations • Loss of depth perception • Inability to determine self-positioning	• Approach from the front. • Use eye contact. • Be reassuring. • Use slow movements. • Guide client. • Maintain safety.
Hippocampus	• Short-term memory • Storage of new memories as long-term memories • Learning	• Has short-term memory loss • Asks repetitive questions • Gets easily confused • Misplaces items • Loses track of time	• Reassure/validate. • Answer questions repeatedly. • Redirect. • Allow time for adjustment.
Amygdala	• Control of flight or fight responses • Emotions • Sexual behavior	• Anger • Inappropriate sexual behavior • Fear	• Distract the client. • Redirect with activities. • Be reassuring.

Handout **1-2**

A Day in the Life of Pat: A Real-Life Scenario

Pat is a 72-year-old retired schoolteacher who lives alone. Pat is having increasing trouble completing the routine of grocery shopping. Pat complains to the store manager about the frequent changes in food placement and even accuses him of hiding the bathroom tissue. The store clerk helps Pat count the money needed to pay for the items. On one occasion, Pat wandered for over one hour in the parking lot looking for the car. When Pat's daughter arrived at the home she found the entire guest room filled with bathroom tissue and no food in the pantry. When confronted, Pat becomes angry and is unable to verbalize any thoughts.

1. List the possible warning signs for Alzheimer's disease, which Pat may be experiencing.

2. Pat's daughter contacted the primary physician for a diagnostic evaluation. What does a diagnostic evaluation include?

3. According to the Global Deterioration Scale (GDS), what stage of Alzheimer's is Pat experiencing?

Handout **1-3**

MODULE 1 UNDERSTANDING DEMENTIA

Causes of Dementia

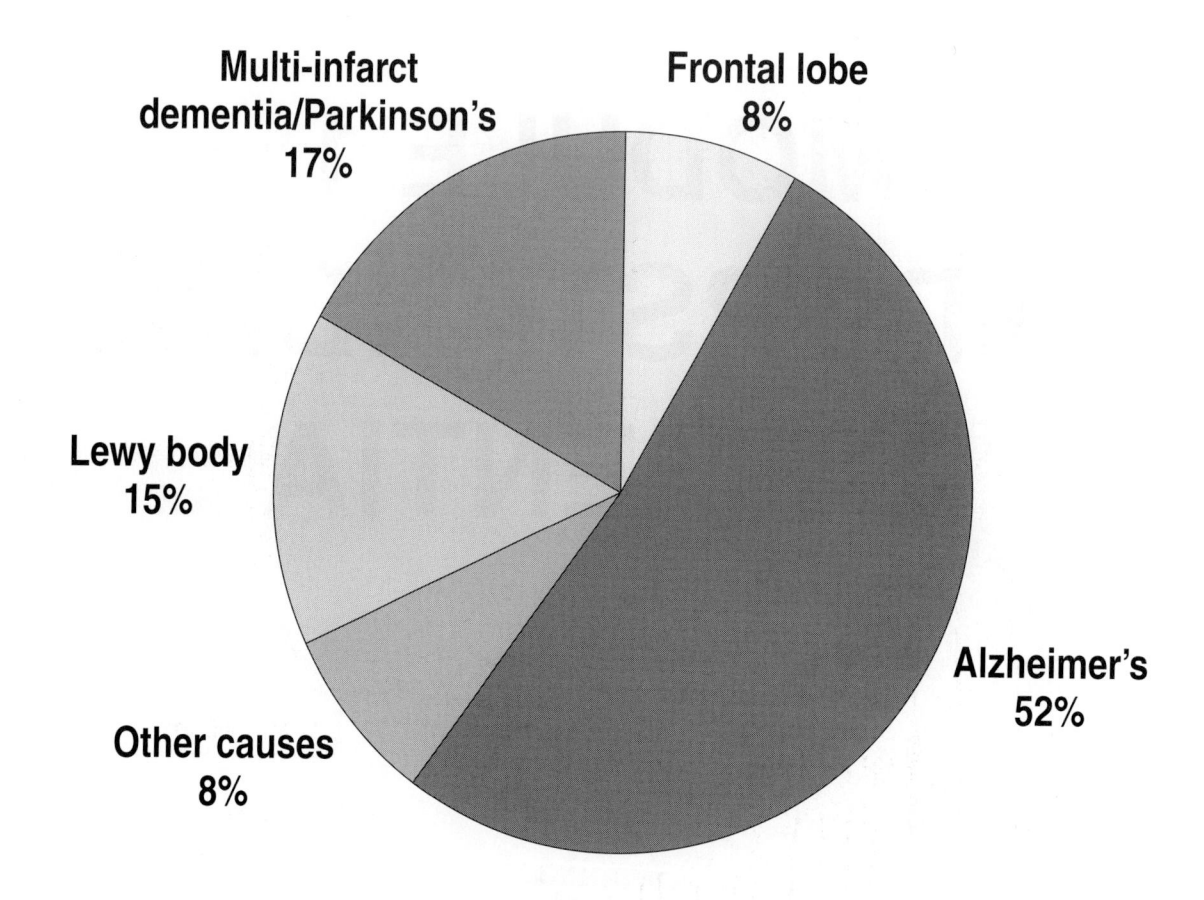

- Multi-infarct dementia/Parkinson's 17%
- Frontal lobe 8%
- Lewy body 15%
- Other causes 8%
- Alzheimer's 52%

Module 1 **UNDERSTANDING DEMENTIA**

The Human Brain

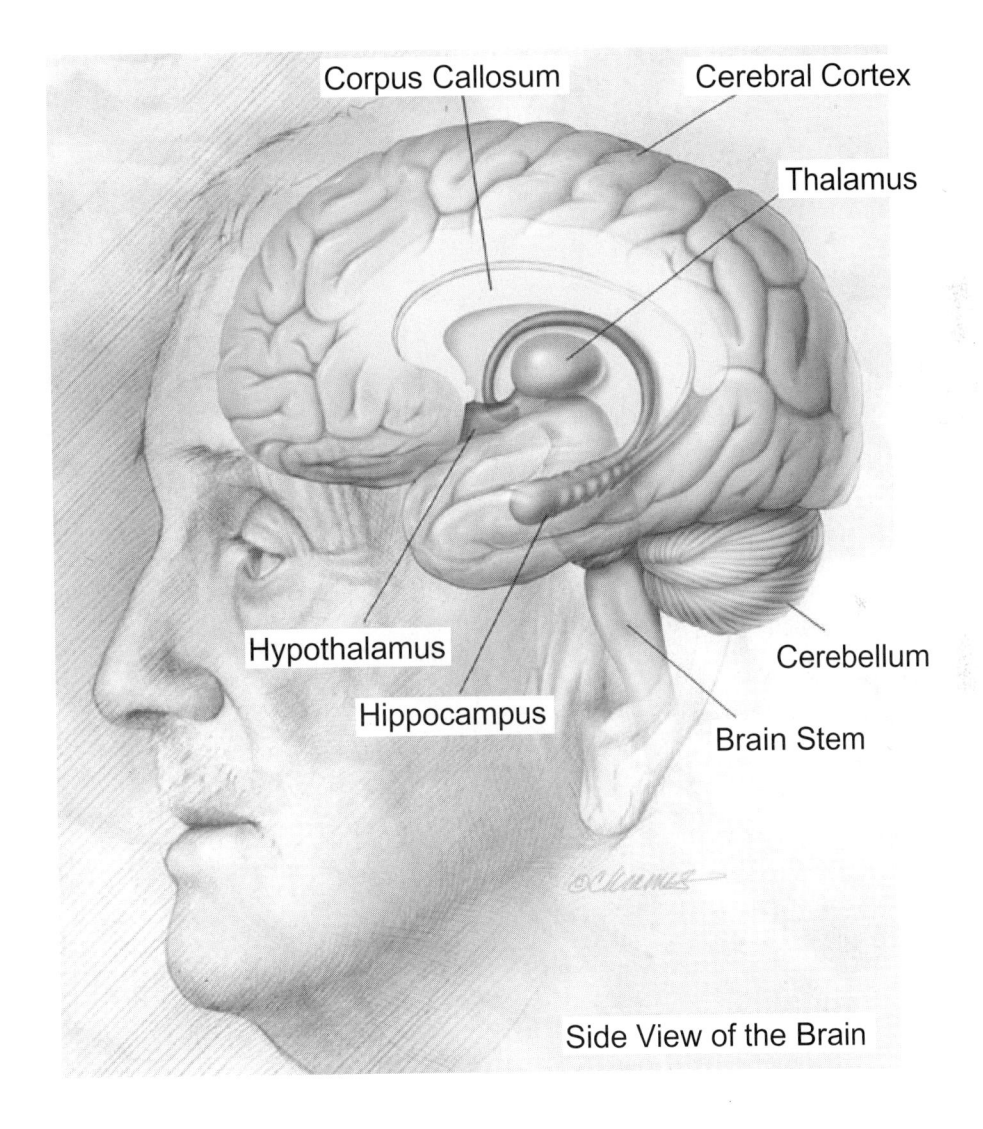

Courtesy of The National Institute on Aging

- Corpus Callosum
- Cerebral Cortex
- Thalamus
- Hypothalamus
- Hippocampus
- Cerebellum
- Brain Stem

Side View of the Brain

Transparency Master **1-3**

Neurons

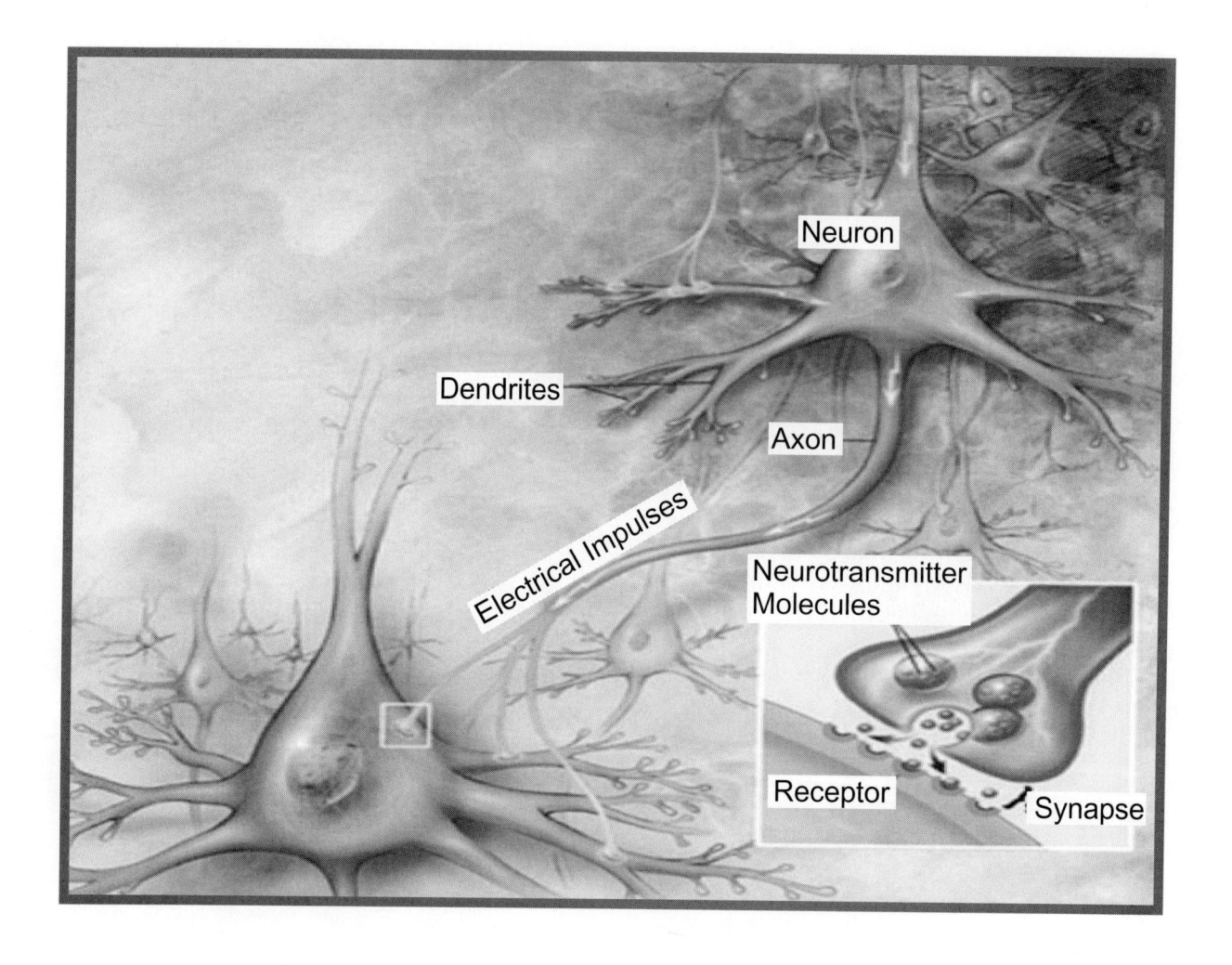

Courtesy of The National Institute on Aging

Beta-amyloid Plaques

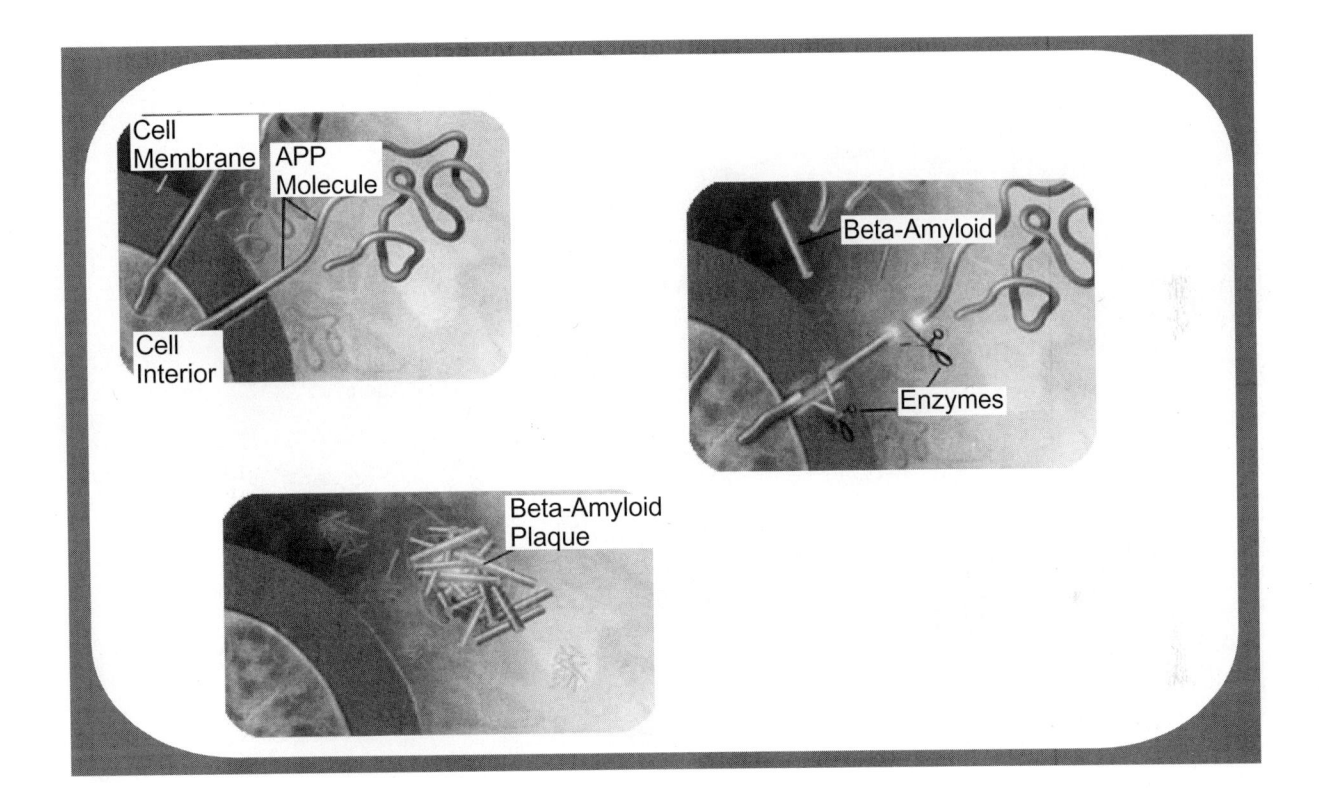

Courtesy of The National Institute on Aging

Neurofibrillary Tangles

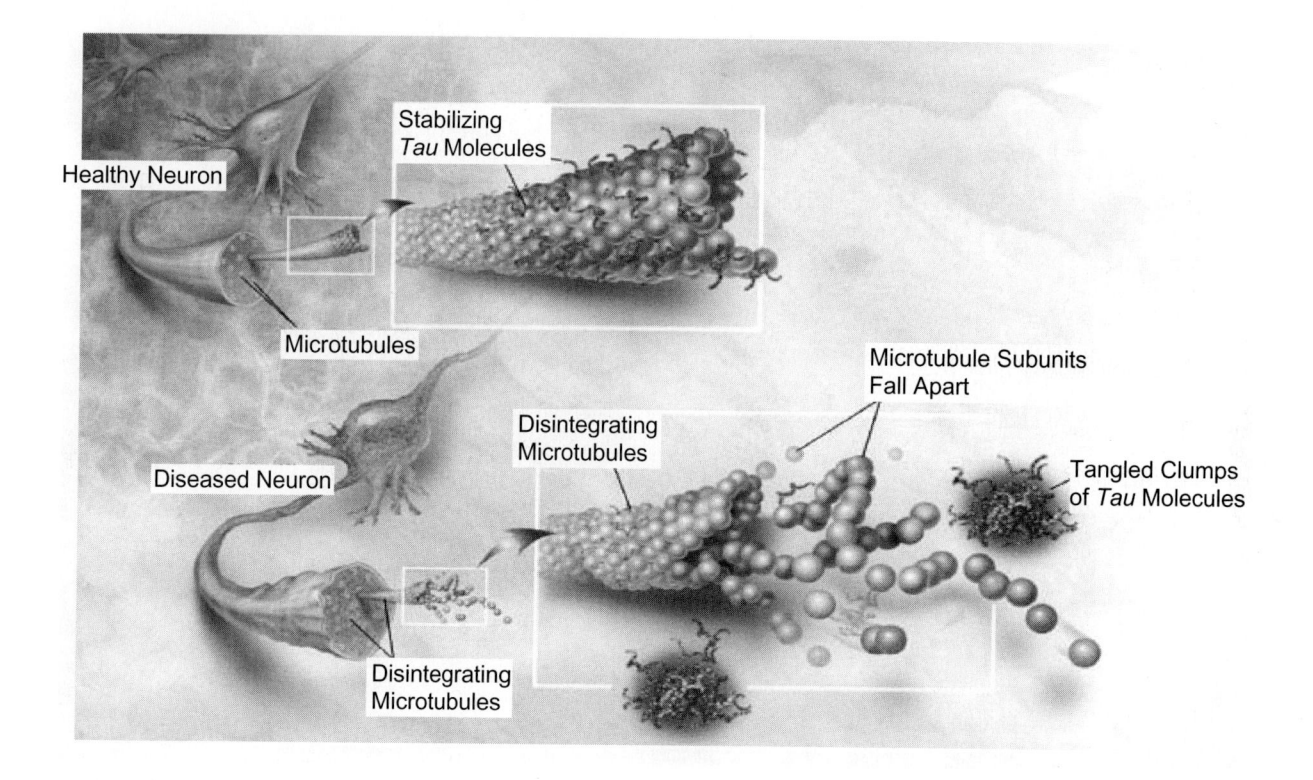

Courtesy of The National Institute on Aging

Cerebral Functions

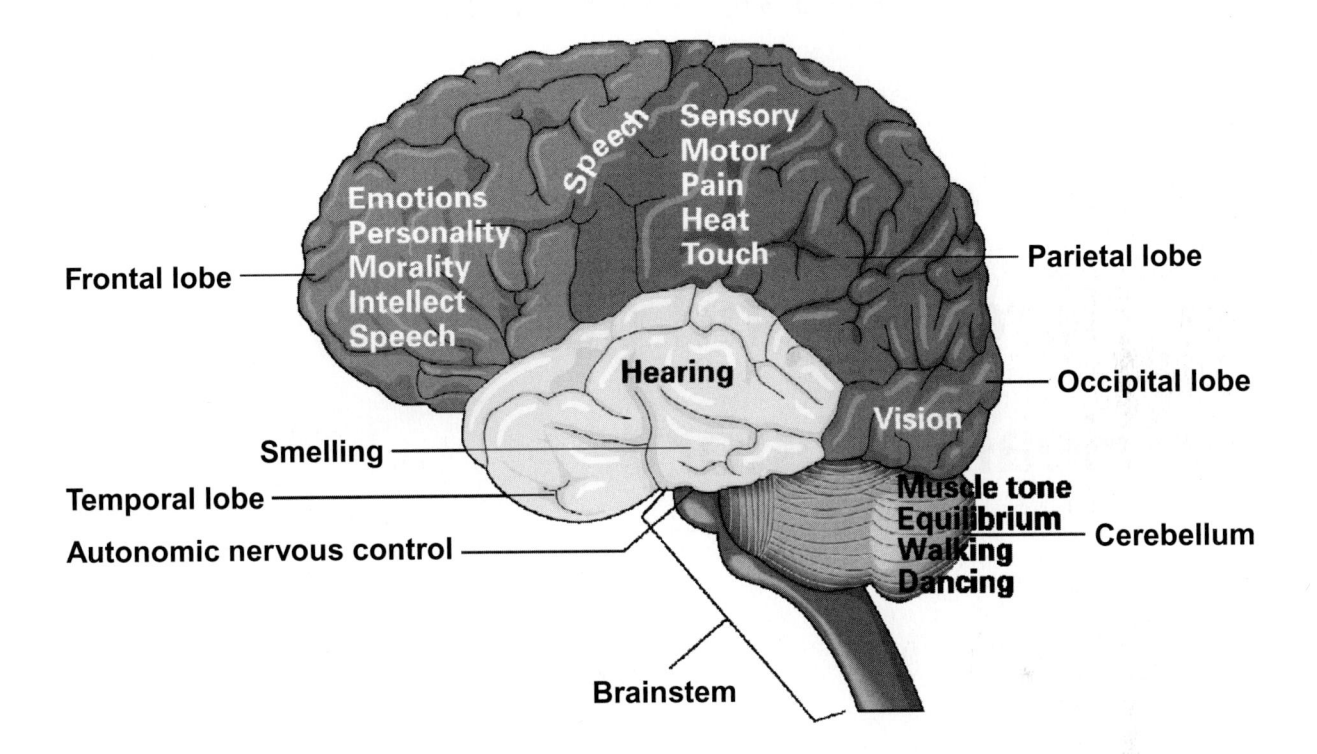

Frontal lobe
- Emotions
- Personality
- Morality
- Intellect
- Speech

Speech

Sensory
Motor
Pain
Heat
Touch

Parietal lobe

Hearing

Occipital lobe

Vision

Smelling

Temporal lobe

Autonomic nervous control

Muscle tone
Equilibrium
Walking
Dancing

Cerebellum

Brainstem

Factors Increasing the Risk for AD

- **Aging**
- **Heredity and genetics**
- **Health history**

Warning Signs of Dementia

- **Forgetfulness**
- **Difficulty with tasks**
- **Language problems**
- **Poor judgment**

Warning Signs of Dementia (*cont.*)

- **Problems with abstract thinking**
- **Misplacing items**
- **Mood/personality/behavioral changes**
- **Loss in initiative**

Diagnostic Evaluation

- **Complete history & physical exam**
- **Psychiatric evaluation**
- **Psychometric testing**

Diagnosing AD

- **Possible AD**
- **Probable AD**
- **Definite AD**

Stages of Alzheimer's Disease

Stage 1 No cognitive decline (normal adult)

Stage 2 Very mild cognitive decline
- aware of function decline
- forgetfulness

Stages of AD

Stage 3 Mild cognitive decline

- becomes lost when traveling
- reduced work performance
- unable to retain written material
- difficulty remembering new people/places

Stages of AD

Stage 4 Moderate cognitive decline

Early stage of AD
- decreased knowledge of current event
- forgets personal history
- decreased concentration

Stages of AD

Stage 5 Moderate severe cognitive decline

- unable to recall major aspects of life
- disoriented to time and place

Stages of AD

Stage 6 Severe cognitive decline

Moderate stage of AD
- **requires assistance with ADL**
- **unable to recall recent events**
- **loss of initiative**
- **obsessive symptoms**

Stages of AD

Stage 7 Very severe cognitive decline

Late stage AD
- unable to perform ADLs
- loss of psychomotor/ communication skills
- death

Treatment Outcomes in AD

- **Maintenance of function**
  - improving symptoms
  - behavioral management
  - family support
- **Slowing the progression of the disease**
- **Prevention/Cure**

Observation and Reporting

How to Report Changes

- **Objective reporting**
- **Subjective reporting**
- **Intuitions**

Module 2
Basic Principles of Dementia Care

Goal
To understand the basic principles of dementia care.

Objectives
After completion of the presentation, students will be able to:
- List the three major aspects of a care plan for a client with dementia.
- Describe the importance of routines for a dementia client.
- Describe breakdowns in the communication process.
- List four common behavioral problems.
- Define the person-centered approach.
- Describe a catastrophic reaction and how should it be approached.

● GENERAL INFORMATION/OVERVIEW

Lecture Material for Slide 1-1

As the population in America ages, the rate of Alzheimer's disease (AD) and other related conditions will steadily increase. Presently, an estimated 4.5 million people have AD. Half of all nursing home residents suffer from Alzheimer's disease or other forms of dementia. Dementia symptoms include the loss of mental faculties relating to memory, personality, and behavior. Caring for such clients becomes a challenge, since many have lost their problem-solving abilities. In addition, behaviors such as confusion, wandering, and agitation need to be part of the care plan focus.

- Managing the behavioral and psychological signs of dementia is a major problem for the health care team. Medications used to treat problem behaviors have a high risk of adverse reactions.

- Dementia symptoms associated with behavioral disturbances may lead to a full spectrum of problems from the trivial to the life threatening. Acute behavioral disturbances for clients with AD often result in emergency room visits and are the most common cause for institutional placement.

- Many methods have surfaced on how to manage a person with dementia, including Montessori-based programming, space-retrieval practice, and validation therapy.

- As the disease progresses, AD clients lose the ability to engage in conversation. Studies show the lack of self-awareness and personal identity lead to physical deterioration and a vegetative state.

- Each client is unique and caregivers should attempt to connect with the person within. Improving quality of life for cognitively impaired individuals is achieved by understanding the person behind the dementia.

● DEVELOPING A PLAN OF CARE

Lecture Material for Slide 2-2

During any stage of the disease, maximizing and maintaining both cognitive and functional abilities are crucial to quality of life. The cognitive deficit of the client with AD poses several challenges to developing a plan. The client should be encouraged to participate in planning, but expectations of self-care should match each client's abilities. Interviewing family members allows the staff to learn about the client's background when the client is unable to fully communicate.

Goals are based on maximizing clients' current abilities and preventing deterioration. Within the plan of care, goals are developed based on modifying their physical and social environment. This maximizes their capabilities and minimizes stressors. Information provided by families enables health care providers to formulate patient-directed care or a person-centered approach. The interventions are based on the client's past experiences, hobbies, and personality. When family is unavailable, utilize the medical record to gather personal aspects about the individual.

Knowing a person's life story, likes, dislikes, and traditions enhances all aspects of Alzheimer's care. Using a person-centered approach makes the difference between a combative client and one who is a joy to be around.

Since each client is unique, not all suggestions can be universally applied. Do not generalize when developing a care plan for a client with AD: "if you have seen one Alzheimer's client, you have seen *one* Alzheimer's client."

Maintaining Physical Health

Monitoring the client's food and fluid intake, bathing, toileting schedule, and sleep routine enables the health care team to improve client care. In comparison to other clients, supporting physical health for a dementia client requires more stringent observation and reporting.

- The alteration in memory is the impetus for diligent caregiver observation and reporting. Changes should be reported to the supervisor to prevent complications, hospitalization, and even death.

- Any safety concerns for the client's activities of daily living are observed and reported to the supervisor immediately. As the client's cognitive abilities change, so do the interventional strategies used for support. Overlooking deficiencies in ADL performance can lead to high-risk outcomes such as dehydration, bowel obstruction, infection, or behavioral problems.

- Observing the client during the daily regimen can identify new physical problems before they become unmanageable. Changes in behavior can be a cue to an underlying illness, such as a urinary track infection. Clients who are unable to communicate their symptoms may use a nonverbal exchange to express their discomfort.

- Changes in sensory perception may also lead to behavioral changes. If the client has changes in communication patterns, ignores stimuli, or withdraws from the environment, assess visual or auditory acuity.

For additional information regarding physical care, see Module 3 and Module 4.

Maintaining a Supportive Physical Environment

Caring for the dementia client includes structuring the environment and activities in ways to compensate for the cognitive loss. The client feels more secure when routines are established and sustained.

- Once the client becomes acclimated to the new environment, change should be kept to a minimum. A regular routine enables the client to know what to expect. Change a routine only when it is no longer working for the client. Clients in the early stages of their illness can adapt to modifications when appropriate.

- The client should stay in the same room, with the same roommate and the same staff, whenever possible. Consistency in the staff assignment benefits the client.

- Families may want to change something in the client's room, such as moving the client's bed near the window. Such changes create a tremendous amount of confusion and anxiety. Environmental changes should occur only when they mimic pre-illness habits.
- Developing a fixed timetable or daily routine, including awakening, toileting, exercise, and meals, gives the client a sense of security.
- The environment should be structured to provide cues for important destinations.
- Areas should have signs with illustrations to help clients gain orientation to their location.
- Using personal items may help clients identify the unfamiliar room as their own.
- Contrasting colors should be used to differentiate perimeters.
- Structure the day so clients are visible to the staff. Numerous mishaps occur when clients are left alone.
- A digital clock, calendar, and a bulletin board should be posted for clients to keep track of time and important messages. Since these abilities are likely to decline with time, adjustments must be made accordingly.
- The environment should remain calm. Surroundings should have little stimulation or confusion. The cognitive deficits limit a person's ability to store ideas simultaneously. Too much noise creates information overload, possibly triggering behavioral problems. Noise should be kept low, and music can be used to mask other extrinsic sounds.

Maintaining a Supportive Social Environment

The approach to interacting with clients is to treat them with respect and dignity. Labeling clients by their behaviors is inappropriate. For example, referring to a client as a "screamer," "a troublemaker," or even by the illness ("the MS client in room 222") promotes staff to think of the client as an obstacle, not a person. Clients whose conduct is troublesome tend to be avoided by the staff, especially dementia clients.

- Research suggests that clients in the middle and late stages of Alzheimer's have some awareness of self. Think of the uniqueness of each Alzheimer's client and how no two clients react alike. Failure by the staff to recognize a client's self-awareness and the human experience can lead to a client's withdrawal and isolation.
- All human beings, including those with memory and cognitive deficiencies, have basic needs: the need to be loved, the need to be useful, and the need to express feelings. Consider the needs of the whole person, which encompass social support, psychological, and physical needs. Incorporate the client's spirituality into the plan of care. The presence of difficult behaviors may be triggered by the caregiver's inability to meet one of the individual's basic needs.
- Activities need to provide meaning and purpose. Much of life that is of value relates to the sense of self and interactions with others. Likes and

dislikes can be acknowledged when disclosed by families. Mr. Smith routinely becomes anxious during bingo, but, after interviewing the family, the staff learns he never enjoyed playing the game.
- Plan appropriate activities that take into account the individual's interest and traditions. Using behavioral and memory interventions helps the client achieve basic humanity.

Lecture Material for Slide 2-3

BEHAVIORAL AND MEMORY INTERVENTIONS

Utilizing strategies to improve behavior and memory can allow the client to function at their highest level of mental and physical capacity.

Task Breakdown Technique

Task breakdown technique is the process of guiding the client through a task while allowing independence and promoting self-esteem.

- The caregiver breaks the task into simplified steps that are manageable for the client. During each incremental step, the client may need prompting or cues.
- At times the caregiver may need to complete the task.
- Praise and reassurance are offered during the process.
- Allow enough time for clients to respond, and repeat instructions if necessary. Use affirmations to remind them of what they should be doing: "Yes, put your socks on first. Uh-huh, the sock goes this way, that's it, almost done. Good job." Always compliment the client's willingness to try.

Montessori-Based Activities

Cameron J. Camp, PhD, director of the Myers Research Institute, utilized the principles of Montessori education; developed by physician and educator Maria Montessori, as an approach to find meaningful activities for clients with dementia.

- The technique allows for the client to successfully complete challenging and intellectual activities. The activities tap into the client's remaining abilities, utilizing the person's procedural memory or implicit memory. Procedural or implicit memory is a memory for information without conscious retrieval. Once an action is learned, the task is completed without consciously retrieving the knowledge to complete the action, for example, walking. This function of the brain remains intact even in the later stages.
- Montessori activities have no final end point and are not childish or just busywork. Activities provide meaningful stimulation as well as guidance in completing tasks successfully.
- The activities center on the client's personal life; if the client was a carpenter by trade, activities should include wood and tools according to the degree of cognitive ability. For example, at first the client may help put together a cabinet, but later in the disease process he or she

may be capable only of sanding a piece of wood. The activity matches the individual person and is worthwhile to the client.
- Successfully performing a challenging and meaningful activity allows clients to feel proud and value the experience, no matter what their stage of dementia.

Space-Retrieval Practice

Camp also developed additional methods to improve memory skills by utilizing the client's preserved memory or procedural memory. He observed dementia clients in the long-term care facility who became agitated when another resident was in their usual seat in the dining hall. Since the facility was not part of their past, the ritual of that seat was learned since their placement. The client may not remember learning it or who taught them, but the memory remains.

- The method begins with asking the person to perform an achievable task. In short intervals of time, repeat the cue to prompt the recollection of the desired behavior. Once this is accomplished, the period between giving the information and asking the person to repeat the behavior is gradually increased. The time between hearing or seeing the information and recall is modified to suit the level of impairment. For example, a person with moderate to severe dementia may be asked to remember something for only a few seconds in the beginning of treatment.
- The practice of space-retrieval can be applied to the basic physical needs of a client. A client was becoming dehydrated because he would not drink. The staff left a glass of water in front of him but he would still not drink. By using space-retrieval, the staff asked the client what was in front of him, and he responded a glass. The staff then replied, "Show me how you drink," and the client drank the water. This was repeated. Now the staff places the glass in front of the client and says, "Drink," and the client does so successfully.
- Success is achieved once the proper cue is determined. Ascertaining the cue requires admission into the world of each dementia client. Grant the client the opportunity to circumvent the disability by promoting success by whatever means necessary.

Validation Therapy

Validation therapy is based on an attitude of respect and empathy for older adults with dementia, developed by Naomi Feil, MSW, ACSW. The intent of the therapy is to accept the values, beliefs, and the reality of the person without proof.

- Validation provides the disoriented person with an empathetic listener, one who is nonjudgmental but accepting of their view of reality. As the trusting relationship grows, the client's anxiety is reduced and his or her sense of self-worth is restored. Validation does not mean lying to or patronizing the client.
- The concept of validation is based on the theory that there is a reason behind all behaviors. Understanding the client's rationale for the

behavior and supporting that need is the key to validation. If clients feel safe, they begin to communicate their true needs.

- The use of validation involves 14 techniques that require no more than eight minutes a day of open, nonjudgmental, empathetic listening. Touch, maintaining eye contact, and matching the client's gestures and emotions are among some of the techniques.

- The following is an example of using validation. A client awakens every night, screaming that there is someone in her room. The staff tries to comfort the client by orienting her to the real world. The client becomes more agitated and needs sedation. With validation, the staff asks, "Who was in your room? What did they want? When did you last see them?" Use the client's answers as clues to what is behind the delusions. Continue to ask the client, "Are there nights when someone does not come into your room?" The client may describe the times when family visits or when there are social events at the facility. The need for socialization and feelings of love could trigger the outbursts. Involving the client in more social events should reduce the behavior. According to validation therapy, by identifying the reason for the behavior (in this example, the need for socialization) and addressing the need, the behavior is reduced or eliminated.

Audience Interaction for Slide 2-3

Ask the audience for a volunteer to come to the front of the class. (The instructor could pose as the volunteer as well.) Ask the volunteer to disclose to the class something their classmates do not know, such as a hobby, a favorite type of music, membership in a group, or an enjoyment in telling jokes. Then ask the audience how this information would help them care for the volunteer if he or she were a client with dementia.

Lecture Material for Slide 2-4

THE COMMUNICATION PROCESS

According to scholar Jurgen Ruesch, who stressed the importance of therapeutic communication in promoting psychological health, human communication is a dynamic process that is influenced by the cognitive and physiological conditions of those involved. He identified three elements involved in the communication process: perception, evaluation, and transmission. Perception occurs when the impulse is transmitted to the brain. Evaluation takes place in the brain, where the message is analyzed; it results in a cognitive response that relates to the informational aspect of the message. Transmission begins once the message is evaluated and perceived by the sender. This feedback influences the continued course of the communication cycle. Feedback stimulates the cycle again until one or more participants terminate the conversation.

Dementia and the Communication Process

Reviewing theories of the communication process enables a visual relationship to emerge and serves in finding and correcting communication breakdowns or problems. In the case of Alzheimer's disease and related dementias, the client may have limitations in each of the described elements.

Problems with Perception, Evaluation, and Transmission

- The initial phase of the process involves getting the client to perceive the original message from the sender. The dementia client may have receptive aphasia (language is not understood), which blocks the process of evaluating the message or content of the information. The client may also have expressive aphasia, that is, words (especially nouns) cannot be formed or expressed.

- Words like "things" or "stuff" might be used more frequently than words specifying an exact idea. The client may have difficulty recalling the names of objects or anomia. The damage to the temporal lobes inhibits memories for words and names, as well as causing disruption in memories for pictures and faces.

- Clients may experience dysarthria, a weakness in the speech muscles due to neurologic damage caused by strokes, illness, or injury, inhibiting transmission of language to the other party. A comorbid condition, such as hearing loss and/or visual disturbance, may also break down communication. Facial expression and body language are unconsciously interpreted as part of the communication process.

- Any condition affecting the client's energy level will interfere in communication. Fatigue, depression, and the side effects of medication play a role in a client's ability to participate in a conversation. Loss of balance and movement may make it difficult for clients to participate in activities and discussions. The client focuses more on maintaining balance and not falling than on the conversation. Also, the limited movement may hinder the client from turning and facing the speaker, missing the message all together.

- The impaired memory may lead the person to unknowingly repeat statements or questions. Losing track of conversations may also be noticeable. Clients may complain that the conversation is moving too fast to understand. The disease not only affects memory and comprehension necessary for communication but also damages speech, language, and social skills needed for a conversation. Clients in the middle stages of the disease cannot see other points of views. They ask fewer questions and make less eye contact. They withdraw from social situations because they have lost the ability to understand prolonged conversation.

- Engaging in conversation, which might have been a simple task before the onset of the disease, now requires more effort. Vocabulary becomes more limited and the ability to process what is said also takes longer. Others participants in the conversation must assume a more active role in compensating for limitations.

Lecture Material for Slide 2-5

COMMON COMMUNICATION CHARACTERISTICS AMONG CLIENTS WITH ALZHEIMER'S DISEASE

- Verbal stereotypic language is characteristic of Alzheimer's disease. Phrases such as "Easier said than done" or "You got me?" are said over and over again. This is a very restricted form of expression and is used as if it were the only language form available.

- The client may speak in generalizations or empty speech. Sentences lack whom, what, or where, and are replaced with general terms. For example, the Alzheimer's client may say, "Here, move this thing over there" instead of "Please put my scarf in the drawer."

- Paraphasias is when an incorrect word is substituted for another. Phonemic paraphasias is when the chosen word sounds similar to the correct word and the message can be understood (eg, pike/pipe, sues/shoes.) Clients with Alzheimer's disease frequently confuse semantically related words or verbal paraphasias (salt/pepper, hot/cold, new/used) or use made-up words that are not part of the person's language or neologistic paraphasias (binse/rug; gumsp/plate).

- The socially accepted rules of conversation are often not adhered to by AD clients. They may interrupt other conversations, make inappropriate and rude statements, or walk away from the speaker.

- All AD clients experience windows of lucidity or moments when suddenly they remember things or speak clearly about a memory or thought. Family members cherish these few moments.

Lecture Material for Slides 2-6 and 2-7

Slide 2-6

COMMUNICATION ABILITIES PRESERVED IN AD CLIENTS

- Procedural memory is preserved until the later stages of the disease, allowing clients to participate in social rituals. Salutations, such as "How are you today?" "Please," and "Thank you," assist in formulating small talk among the residence and staff.

- Clients with dementia have the ability to access early life memories. Encourage family and staff to discuss childhood memories with the clients. The memories are easier for the client to recall, limiting frustration and behavioral challenges. This connection helps to satisfy the client's desire for interpersonal communication and respect.

- Clients are able to recite, read aloud, and sing common greetings, prayers, or songs. These activities themselves encourage self-esteem, comfort, and joy. Clients still have the ability to comprehend even after their written and spoken language has been impaired. Playing music and reading to them also foster the same emotions.

- AD clients expect to be treated as adults and react more positively when addressed respectfully. Though their behaviors may mimic those of a child, their years of experiences earned them respect and dignity. "Always treat clients as you would want to be treated."

Nonverbal Communication

Understanding the importance of communication is the foundation for all interactions with people who have AD. The behaviors of AD clients say more about what they are feeling than they can express in words. How they feel about themselves, how comfortable they are in a situation and surroundings, or how anxious they are with others can be assessed with nonverbal communication.

- Nonverbal communication includes everything that does not involve the spoken or written word: body language (posture and position), tones of voice, gestures, facial expressions, touch, and eye contact.
- This level of communication is often unconsciously motivated and may more accurately indicate a person's meaning than the words being used.
- When increased anxiety or other behavioral changes occur, observe all verbal and nonverbal messages.

Conversational Techniques

- Maintain a calm and pleasant approach. Any personal emotions need to be neutralized before speaking with the client; be nonjudgmental. The person with dementia will mirror your mood.
- The success or failure of a conversation rests heavily on the staff's communication skills. Tone of voice, listening skills, biases, and cultural and linguistic differences all influence communication.
- Due to the damage to the occipital lobe of the brain in clients with AD, always approach the client from the front. Do not start a conversation while approaching them; first establish eye contact. Speak at their eye level whenever possible, sit next to them on the sofa, or bend down to meet their eyes.
- Use gentle touch to calm and reassure the person. Physical touch may frighten some clients; so observe for any behavioral changes and act accordingly.
- When talking with Alzheimer's disease clients, use questions that offer choices, such as, "Do you want to wear the red shirt or the blue one?" Most often the later choice is requested because it is the last word heard by the client. The use of open-ended questions may lead to frustration or no response, ending the conversation. Eliminate any distractions; for example, shut the client's door if the hallways are noisy or shut off the television.
- Asking yes or no questions is appropriate when stimulating conversation is not necessary. Yes or no answers allow clients to communicate their needs without much effort. Speak slowly and use short simple sentences.

Slide 2-7

- Stimulating conversation may require the staff to start a sentence and let the client finish. The technique of closure helps a client respond to familiar expressions by using the procedural memories that stay intact. Examples are "Your husband's name is . . ." and "Do you want a piece of . . . ," while pointing to the cake. Words remain longer in the client's vocabulary the more often they are used.
- Assist the client with word searching. Correct or repair the client's statement by editing the mistaken word without criticizing. If the client says, "It is snowing," reply with the corrected word while validating his or her commitment to the conversation: "Yes it is

raining, the river is very high." Include the nouns or missing words that the client may omit during the conversation (anomia): "It is over there" would be replaced with a statement such as "Yes, your shoes are in the closet." The client may correct the statement if it is inaccurate.

- Avoid giving clients orders. Demanding a client do something only creates more resistance. When requiring a client to complete a certain task, describe each step with a short and simple instruction. Gestures, cues, and physical prompts assist the client with understanding the conversation.

Given the right support, clients with Alzheimer's are still capable of having a brief but meaningful conversation. Their attempts to communicate deserve positive acknowledgment. Maintaining all social abilities should be encouraged. Caregivers who respond to clients' efforts in a positive manner protect the client from feelings of worthlessness and despair by fulfilling their basic needs.

BEHAVIORAL CHALLENGES

Lecture Material for Slide 2-8

The effects of Alzheimer's disease are cruel and nondiscriminatory. The progression of cognitive and functional decline is an expected trademark of the disease. The behavioral changes manifested by the disease are not completely anticipated and understood. Persons who lived their lives following the cultural and social norms are now displaying behaviors that conflict with their character. Severe mood swings, verbal or physical aggression, combativeness, repetition of words, and wandering lead to frustration and tension not only for people with AD but also for their caregivers. Always remember persons with AD are unable to control their behavior and that their actions are never planned.

Audience Interaction for Slide 2-8

Ask the audience, "What does a behavior mean?"

The discussion should focus on how a behavior, whether good or bad, is a form of communication and has a purpose. The act itself is not intended to annoy or torment anyone.

Common Causes of Behavioral Changes

Any behavior exhibited by clients with AD has a purpose. Think of their behavioral changes as a secret language, which they may or may not understand. Persons with AD *do not* act this way on purpose. The damage to the brain, especially to the amygdala, frontal lobe, and temporal lobes, are thought to be the cause. Physical and social environments also play a role in these unwanted behaviors. The occurrence of the behaviors is individual to each AD client. Family involvement is crucial for identifying treatable behaviors, recreating behavioral history, and monitoring changes.

Physical Discomfort

- Behavioral changes can be the result of an illness or medication, such as a urinary tract infection.
- Clients who are unable to communicate their symptoms may use a nonverbal exchange to express their discomfort.
- Observe and report all behaviors to the supervisor in order to treat discomforts and medical conditions.

Lack of Recognition

- The world around AD clients changes faster than they can interpret. Family members may appear as potential threats. Their surroundings are strange and unfamiliar.
- Many clients are looking for their childhood homes and living in their earlier life.
- Interventions of calming memories may help. Use reminiscing, personal photographs, and validate any fears to distract and console clients.

Overstimulation

- Loud noise or too much stimulation confuses the already disoriented Alzheimer's client.
- The brain no longer is able to translate input from different sources concurrently.
- Introduce one issue or one instruction at a time to allow clients the chance to filter and understand the information. When they can focus on one thing, filter the information, and understand it, the environment becomes more controlled and less overwhelming.

Difficulty Completing Simple Tasks or Activities

- With the progression of the illness, once obtainable goals become frustrating and impossible.
- Many times clients are aware they no longer can complete the multitasked duties of their past.
- Use techniques such as Montessori-based activities, space-retrieval methods, and a person-centered approach to minimize client frustrations.

Inability to Communicate Effectively

- One basic human need is to express feelings.
- Experts believe all types of behavior are forms of communication. Communications skills are greatly affected in AD clients.

Audience Interaction for Slide 2-8

Ask the audience how observation and reporting can help the client with a behavioral change.

Lecture Material for Slide 2-9

● EXPLORING CAUSES AND SOLUTIONS TO BEHAVIORAL CHANGES

Since all behaviors are forms of communication and have meaning, decoding what the AD client is trying to express is an important social need. Dementia clients no longer have the ability to follow logic; so it can be exhausting for caregivers to determine what the behavior means. The actions or interventions to diminish such behaviors should be based on the nature of the behavior or type of behavior.

Types of Behaviors

- Common behaviors (eg, repetitive behaviors) are more of an annoyance than a problem and should not lead to an argument with the client.
- Challenging behaviors (eg, shouting, elopements) are behaviors that can lead to more troublesome events if not intervened by the caregiver. Interventions should be swift to avoid further problems.
- Harmful behaviors (eg, violence, hitting) are behaviors that have the potential to cause harm or that do cause harm to the clients or others. Take necessary actions to eliminate the damaging behavior.

Identify the Behavior

By identifying the behavior, the health care team can try to determine purpose. Find the who, what, where, when, and why of the behavior.

- What is the change in behavior?
- Is the behavior harmful to the client or to others?
- Does the behavior violate the rights of others?
- Does the behavior make it difficult to care for the needs of the client?
- What happened prior to the behavior occurring?
- When did the behavior occur?
- Where does the behavior occur?
- Why did the behavior start?
- How did the behavior begin? Did something trigger it?
- Is the behavior a reaction to a new medication?

Explore Potential Solutions

- Everything surrounding a person could contribute to the behavior problem: noise, crowds, and lighting. Is there something in the environment causing the behavior? Does the client need or want something?
- Clients mimic the emotions of those around them. Acknowledge the client behavior in a calm and supportive way. How is the caregiver responding?

- Remove and avoid all triggers that provoke a challenging behavior.
- Psychosocial interventions facilitate better practical management and can evoke key responses from the client's subconscious.
- Unless symptoms are reckless, monitoring the behavior for at least one month should be considered before starting medications.

Alternative Approaches

- Since the caregiver may not know the underlying reason for the behavior, modifications in the approach may be necessary. Solutions may change daily and varied approaches may be needed. If one intervention did not work, leave the client and return in about 10 minutes. The client's short-term memory loss allows for a new creative approach without judgments or resentment over previous attempts.
- Acknowledge clients' requests and respond. Validate their feelings. Try to evoke conversation to allow them to express their needs. Tailor the approach to their functioning level.
- Share solutions with others members of the health care team. Interview family members for cues of behaviors.
- The importance of observation and reporting cannot be overemphasized. Be alert to the environment and all behaviors. Observing clients' interactions with residents and/or the environment can provide for cues on what triggers problem behaviors.

Lecture Material for Slides 2-10, 2-11, and 2-12

Slide 2-10

Audience Interaction for Slides 2-10, 2-11, and 2-12

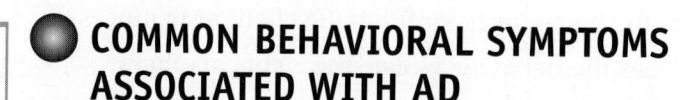

COMMON BEHAVIORAL SYMPTOMS ASSOCIATED WITH AD

Although dementia produces certain kinds of behaviors, some behaviors may be more or less regulated according to the nature of the environment, routines, and interactions with others. The following discussion reviews behavioral symptoms commonly observed in clients with Alzheimer's disease.

Ask the audience to name common behavioral symptoms associated with AD.

Apathy

- Apathy and indifference are the most common behavioral symptoms associated with AD. Clients have a reduced interest in activities. An apathetic client lacks emotions, motivation, interest, and enthusiasm. The behavioral change presents itself early in the disease.
- Apathy is not depression, though 10% of AD clients suffer from major depression. The client is unmotivated and does not have the ability to "get up and go." The damage to the frontal lobe, which is responsible for the ability to initiate activity, may be the cause.

- Though AD clients' affect appears calm, withdrawing from their environment only heightens their isolation. Encourage clients to participate in activities; talk to them about their hobbies and interests. Forcing them to participate may trigger a catastrophic reaction; so pace the interaction accordingly.
- If clients take part in the activity for only a few moments, praise them on what they accomplished and reinforce the behavior. Slowly lengthen the time of the activity each day.

Anxiety

- The fact that people with Alzheimer's disease are anxious should not be a surprise to anyone. Misplacing items and being unable to find them, not recognizing friends and family, and forgetting how to get home may elicit panic. Changes in the brain, which affect emotions and coping skills, increase apprehension. Anxiety can also be contributed to medications, physical and social environments, and coexisting illnesses.
- Anxiety may provoke other behaviors, such as restlessness, pacing, repeating of questions, or other repetitive activities.
- Depending on the client's symptoms, pharmaceutical intervention may help. Again, with any drug regime, use of medications should be based on individual needs.

Agitation

- "Agitation" is a term used to describe behaviors such as screaming, shouting, complaining, moaning, cursing, pacing, fidgeting, and even wandering.
- Clients may become agitated if they are in pain, anxious, fearful, or overwhelmed, or if anything interferes with their ability to think clearly. Do not try to rationalize why they are feeling this way; most of the time such behaviors are misdirected and exaggerated.
- The client may not be angry at all. The emotion is most likely due to a misinterpretation of the conversation or surroundings.
- When a change in the client's behavior (agitation or screaming) occurs, first rule out a medical cause. AD clients may not be able to express their symptoms and so they act out.
- Do not respond to the anger. Try to ignore the negative behaviors whenever possible and reward positive behaviors.
- Try to identify what triggers the agitation. Changing the environment or the caregiver, as well as just simplifying the routines, may ease agitation. Distract agitated clients and redirect their attention. Reduce unnecessary stimuli. Use calm, soft tones and positive statements.
- When physical or verbal aggression intensifies, the caregiver should step back and try to distract the individual. When safety becomes an issue, antipsychotic medications may be tried.

- Anger and violent behaviors are part of a catastrophic reaction and should be handled accordingly. (Catastrophic reactions will be discussed in detail later in the module.) Eliminating the exacerbation of the behavior and preventing the episode altogether is more appropriate. Restraints and sedatives should be used judiciously.

Combativeness

- Combativeness includes words, lashing out, agitation, and it may lead to physical violence. Clients who feel frustrated or pressured to complete a task may become combative and push the caregiver.
- Clients may be fatigued, overstimulated, or may have an adverse reaction to a medication.
- To better support clients and those around them, intervene at the first sign of frustration and avoid a combative episode. Use a calming voice and redirect the client to a simpler task. Observe their level of function and report any changes in order for the plan of care to be adjusted.
- Successful communication can reduce frustration. Clear, simple statements with gestures enable the client to better understand how to succeed at the task. Limiting choices empowers clients to make decisions without feeling frustrated and anxious.
- As with any behavioral symptom, do not argue or force the client to complete the activity.

Slide 2-11

Repetitive Behaviors

- Repetitive behaviors are activities, questions, outbursts, and stories executed over and over again. Persistent repetition is also known as perseveration. Clients who are perseverating may pack and unpack clothing from a drawer (rummaging) for no purpose or repetitively pace up and down the room.
- The action may be related to a former job or activity. The businessperson may carry a briefcase at all times; the schoolteacher may rearrange the chairs; and the homemaker may repeatedly fold the clothes.
- Asking questions repetitively results from the memory loss of asking the question or of hearing the answer. Clients may feel insecure or anxious, feelings that may play a part in their repetitive questioning. Calmly answer the question twice, once for communication and once for the client. Discovering the reason for the behavior is the way to find solutions. If the client is continually asking to go home (meaning the childhood home) respond by inquiring about the place she grew up: "What color was your house?" or "What was the best thing about it?"
- The lack of activity and boredom contribute to repetitive behaviors. Find activities that stimulate the client and provide social contact. Activities should be client-centered and reflect something they value.

- If the repetitive questioning is due to memory loss, list or use visual aids to help stimulate memories. Have a daily schedule posted so clients can be reminded of the day's activities.
- Shadowing is when a client follows or mimics the caregiver. Clinging behavior can be noted in an overwhelming situation. The behavior may be triggered by agitation. To avoid shadowing, replace the behavior with successful activities, notably promoting self-esteem and keeping the client occupied. Stuffing envelopes, folding towels, or listening to music can be instrumental in reducing the behavior. Taking a few minutes a day and dedicating them to communicating with the client can reduce the person's loneliness, which is being expressed through the repetitive behaviors. Never underestimate how important personal attention is to the client. Support groups and group meetings are helpful means for reducing shadowing.
- Use touch to redirect the person when being physically repetitive. Stroking an object also helps funnel the behavior. Observe for skin breakdown or physical complaints due to the activity. If the client cannot stop pacing, encourage him or her to have a snack to maintain caloric intake.
- Creative solutions may need to be tested to find success. Try to remain controlled, and take a deep breath before the repetitive behavior returns.

Hoarding

- Hoarding is a common behavior among AD clients and represents cognitive damage. Collecting items, food, or dirty clothes and hiding them in strange locations have a few possible motivations. First, the client may feel insecure and the possessions represent security. Second, the client may not be able to determine what has value. Last, discarding items requires decision-making skills, which are no longer available to the client. Severe hoarding causes safety and health hazards. Clients may not be aware they are hoarding the items.
- The belongings will habitually be hidden in the same place. Routinely check clients' rooms for saved food, dirty clothes, or other possessions. To help diminish anxiety, leave a few of the items, provided the material will not spoil or attract insects. Food should be kept in a closed container. Frequently remind the client of the location of their "stash" to reduce the taking of additional items.

Wandering

- Wandering can become dangerous when clients leave the safety and security of their home and environment.
- Try to determine whether the wandering seems aimless or has a purpose. Does the client appear to be looking for a misplaced item? Is the client looking for positive stimulation? Does the wandering occur

at the same time? Is the client wandering after a stressful situation or out of fear?

- Approach from the front and guide the client in a more suitable direction. Avoid turning him or her around; this limits confrontation and promotes positive behavior. Reassure the person and minimize additional stressors.

- Try to develop client-directed solutions. Maybe the client has a previous agenda and is "trying" to get to work or retrieve his or her young children from school. (Try to stop an eighty-year-old mother with dementia from attending to her lost children.) Past roles are the client's present reality. Solutions should distract the client from wandering by addressing that role. For example, ask the mother who wanders to tell you about her children. Have a desk with letters and papers near the door, so that the wandering secretary stops and fixes the clutter on the desk. Each example gives the client a purposeful activity.

For detailed lecture material, see Module 5.

Sleep Disturbances

- Changes in sleep patterns are a normal part of aging but can be significantly troublesome for caregivers of dementia clients. Clients with early AD can awaken at night, be extremely confused, and wanting to wander outside or act on some delusion. They may awaken and resume daytime activities, disturbing others.

- Pacing, agitation, wandering, and confusion during the late afternoon and evening hours characterize sundowning, the most common sleep problem. The cause of sundowning is not known. Research suggests the stress of the day and the person's inability to control symptoms due to fatigue trigger the event. Think of how small children react when they do not have their afternoon nap. Try to observe for possible triggers that provoke their behavioral changes. If the client appears fatigued due to the daily routines, incorporate rest periods earlier in the day to minimize fatigue and stress in the evenings.

- Assess clients for factors that contribute to keeping them awake. Observe for pain, medications, fear, noise, and lighting. Subtle changes in the environment may assist the person in reestablishing a normal sleep pattern. A night-light may provide the client with a feeling of security.

- Clients with sleep disturbances should be kept active during the day and should not spend the day resting and napping. Exercise and activities should be planned so the client expends energy and becomes more fatigued at bedtime.

- The establishment of nighttime rituals helps the client identify bedtime. Remember clients feel more secure when routines are established and sustained.

- Incorporate a light snack into the evening routine. Encourage the use of the bathroom before the client retires to bed. Often clients awake to use the bathroom, become disorientated, and panic because they do not recognize the environment during the nighttime hours.

Slide 2-12

Sexual Behavior

- Behaviors, including sexual behavior, undergo significant changes and are usually marked by alteration in the person's demeanor or personality. A small percentage of Alzheimer's type dementia exhibit inappropriate sexual behaviors.

- Clients who are demonstrating an increased demand for sexual gratification should not be labeled as "oversexed," "perverted," or "a dirty old man." Remember the part of the brain (amygdala) that controls sexual behavior is damaged. The person is unable to control sexual hunger.

- Other possible causes of the sexual behaviors can be contributed to external stimuli, prescription medications, or the limited physical gratification the client is able to experience.

- Heightened activity in seeking sexual gratification tends to be associated with restlessness and irritability. Research suggests that changes in sexual behavior can be associated with affect disabilities or mood disorders as well as the person's activity.

- AD clients may misinterpret the actions of others, which can lead to behaviors that appear to be sexually motivated. Male clients may develop an erection when being bathed or become confused by the caregiver's words or actions. Staff may assume a behavior is sexual in nature when it is not. A woman taking off a garment may simply mean she is warm or it is uncomfortable.

- Clients may reach out to other residents for affection and personal contact. Liaisons between residents should be handled with dignity and respect. Discussions regarding appropriateness should include families. Ethical issues arise over whether a person who is impaired can or should make sexual decisions for themselves.

- Problems associated with sexual behaviors include indecent behaviors, sexually explicit behaviors, and sexual harassment. An indecent behavior is a suggestion of sexuality and can include a hug, a more-than-friendly kiss, or a lewd joke.

- Sexually explicit behaviors are often considered distasteful and unpleasant to witness. Possible behaviors may include masturbation and exposing genitalia, which can be embarrassing to family and staff. Explain to bystanders that the client is confused; in most cases, clients forget to dress and are unaware of their nudity. When the behavior takes place publicly, escort the client to a private area.

- Sexual harassment or staff harassment is a sensitive issue. When the sexual behaviors are not warranted and cause the recipient to feel threatened, the behavior is harassment. Interventions should incorporate all involved, including staff and families. Harassment is a very sensitive issue since all parties involved have a valid reason for their actions. The behavior is offensive and victims deserve to feel safe. Dementia clients cannot be held accountable for their actions due to their cognitive loss.

Insert the agency's sexual harassment policy here.

- As with any behavioral change, the need to identify the cause and find solutions remains. Distracting clients and redirecting them to another activity can help.
- Address clients' need for intimacy throughout the day to give them the attention they crave. Intimacy and physical contact can be achieved without sexual connotation. Encourage family members to hold their hands and embrace them during visits.

Uncooperative Behaviors

- Refusing or resisting requests is very troublesome to caregivers. Wanting to provide quality care is the primary objective of all caregivers. The uncooperative client can make anyone less than compassionate. Always remember the behavior is not personal. The refusal is not directed at caregivers or those around them but is part of the disease process.
- Due to the nature of the illness clients may not always understand what is being asked of them. Fear itself may cause resistance, especially when there is a change in the environment.
- Clients may refuse to complete a task simply because of their memory loss. They are unable to remember when they last took a bath and become insulted when told to bathe.
- Make sure the requests are being understood. Use simple sentences, which explains what is needed. If the client refuses to eat the sandwich, try to explain what it is and how to eat it.
- Develop rituals for outings or opposed events. If the client often refuses to go to the doctor, associate the trip with a pleasant experience, such as ice cream, walks in the garden, or a favorite activity. Anything that makes clients feel safe and allows them to cooperate is acceptable.
- Clients who routinely are demanding about everything may have learned that the only way staff or family pays attention to them is by complaining. The underlying need may simply be the need for human contact. Sitting down with each client for a few minutes per week may reduce the unwanted behavior.
- Sometimes nothing convinces the client to cooperate. Also, consider the fact that some people are more uncooperative than others by nature. The client may be too confused to comprehend even his or her own emotions. Avoid arguments and accept whatever compromise works.

Accusations/Suspiciousness/Paranoia

- Suspiciousness is a commonly observed behavior in the latter stages of the disease. The behavior is contributed to a faltering memory and/or an inability to recognize friends and family.
- Fear is usually the underlying reason for all accusations.

- By blaming others, clients distance themselves from what they believe is the problem. For example, the client may blame the roommate for stealing his money, when in fact he put the money away and cannot recall where it is placed. Blaming the roommate lessens the fear experienced regarding the memory loss. Another example is blaming the leaking pipes for the wet bed sheets, when the client becomes incontinent. He is unable to understand, cope, or communicate what is actually happening and blames the wet sheets on something else.

- Determine whether the accusations are true or false. The caregiver needs to protect clients in the event their fears are real. Many times their behaviors go uninvestigated because no one takes them seriously. They may complain that another resident is stealing their food, when in fact the resident does eat the cookies that the family leaves. Another interpretation of the accusations is that the client is hungry and unable to verbalize hunger.

- Paranoid suspicions can escalate to delusions. The belief that someone is trying to hurt or steal from them can cause unpredictable reactions. Studies show 50% of Alzheimer's clients experience paranoid delusions regarding theft or betrayal.

- Do not underestimate the strength of the frail 90-year-old female if she believes she is in danger. The disappearance of cognition, memory, and health make the client feel extremely vulnerable to harm.

- The caregiver's goal is to restore order when suspicious behaviors occur. Whenever there is a confrontation, always be the mediator. Validate the feelings of all involved and use soft-spoken words. The parties involved may imitate the voice and calm demeanor. Reassure the suspicious client and lead him or her away from the area. The accused resident needs reassurance as well. Provide encouragement for all positive responses. Do not scold anyone.

Delusions

- Delusions are very common among clients with AD and contribute to the deterioration of the person's quality of life. Delusions are beliefs that remain fixed in a person's mind despite reasonable evidence.

- Many delusions can be harmless while others play a critical role in institutionalizing clients.

- Clients with cognitive losses are trying to make sense of their past experiences.

- Challenging the delusion only cause Alzheimer's clients to feel threatened and vulnerable "Going along" with the delusion is not appropriate either. Lying to them about the reality does not resolve the real cause of the delusions.

- Try to enter their world. Acknowledge the underlying emotion and redirect their current thinking. If they begin to talk about their dead mother as if she were still alive, respond by saying something about the mother and ask them to talk about her. For example, "Your mother sounds like a kind woman. Can you tell me about her?" Or "What did you like most about her?"

- The caregiver should validate clients' physical and emotional pain and assure them they are safe. As mentioned earlier in the lecture, the concept of validation is based on the theory that there is a reason behind all behaviors. Listening to clients and helping them through the delusion should ease the anxiety associated with it and minimize the frequency.

- The use of antipsychotic drugs should be based on each client's individual needs and not routinely prescribed.

Catastrophic Reaction

- Catastrophic reactions are extreme emotional responses to trivial events causing the person to have sudden mood changes, crying, screaming, or even physical violence.

- The behavior is very typical among AD clients and is most likely due to overstimulation in the environment. The person's decreased capacity to inhibit emotional responses contributes to the intensity of the reaction. Attempting tasks that are too complex or questioning may provoke an event.

- Catastrophic reactions are frightening to both the client and the caregiver.

- Prevention of catastrophic reactions should be a part of the care plan for clients who are more susceptible. Avoiding situations known to trigger the reaction can be achieved with careful planning.

- The use of distraction can be beneficial to clients if they are experiencing excessive emotions. Caregivers should not overreact to the behavior for it has the potential to escalate the catastrophic reaction.

Lecture Material for Handout 2-2

BASIC PRINCIPLES OF CARE

The ideology of the basic principles of care will be utilized in all aspects of dementia care and should be reinforced with each module. This section is designed to review the major content of the lecture. Information can be reinforced through audience interaction or traditional lecture. Have the students use the handout for note taking.

Use Effective Communication Skills

- Use simple sentence structure with only the information the person needs to know. Too many words may distract the person and the message will not be understood.

- Simplify statements to include only one thought. "The doctor's office called and changed your appointment from Friday to today." This statement has far to many thoughts for the AD client to understand quickly. Tell the client he or she has a doctor's appointment today.

Reduce Distractions and Avoid Information Overload

- Limit distracting noises. Lower the television volume; choose quiet places to talk.
- Provide only the amount of information the client can process. Too many choices overwhelm the client and create more confusion. Lay out a few outfits for the client to select rather than having them look through the entire closet for something to wear.

Positively Address Feelings of Insecurity

- Do not argue with the accusatory client. The client's ability to process correcting information has been impaired. Stress this point to family members.
- Validate the client's feelings.
- Encourage the client to be as independent as possible. Give the individual every opportunity to function at maximum potential by helping him or her successfully complete tasks.

Use Message Boards, Signs, or Pictures

- Clients may forget appointments or placement of items but retain the ability to read words or understand pictures. Speech is not the only way to communicate.
- Using any method to help the client successfully perform daily activities will only increase self-esteem and reduce anxiety.

Use Touch

- Touch can provide sensory stimulation, reduce anxiety, and relieve physiological and emotional pain. Use touch to guide a client away from a harmful situation to a more appropriate activity.
- Touch should convey respect and sensitivity for the client.
- Touch is a form of communication. Various messages are conveyed through touch, such as affection, emotional support, encouragement, tenderness, pain, and attention seeking.
- Although touch can be helpful to a client, its use must always be clearly understood and accepted.

Pick "Your" Battles

- Some battles are not worth fighting. If conditions are not harmful to clients or those around them, rescind the request. If the client does not want to take a shower today and is getting increasingly agitated, let it go. If the client has an odor and truly needs to bathe, try again later after the client has rested.

- When a client becomes increasingly agitated and immediate attention is given, the negative behavior is reinforced. Altering the caregiver's reactions prevents reinforcing the negative behavior.
- Set priorities by addressing client's environment, health needs, proper nutrition, reducing medical symptoms, and taking medications.

Do Not Take the Behaviors Personally

- AD clients are unable to comprehend the surrounding world. They unknowingly forget something, thus affecting routines. Be careful not to blame or scold them.
- Any inappropriate behavior is due to the disease, not the person. The client is not acting in that manner on purpose or "to get to you."

Center "Yourself"

- Clients sense feelings and mimic emotions.
- Count to ten before approaching a client when feeling tense.

SUMMING UP

The basic principles of dementia care are meant to help clients maximize both their cognitive and functional abilities. The health care team develops the plan of care, which focuses on three aspects of the client's well-being, supporting their physical health, physical environment, and social environment. The interventions to maintain the goals of the care plan are person-centered and rely on family and friends for insight when the client is unable to participate in the planning process.

Behavioral and memory interventions, such as task-breakdown technique, Montessori-based activities, space-retrieval practices, and validation therapy, assist clients in functioning at their highest level of capacity, enhancing their quality of life. Preserving AD clients' ability to communicate helps acknowledge their needs, wants, and desires. The frequency of challenging behaviors lessens when the reasons behind the unwanted behaviors are discovered and solutions identified.

Module 2 **BASIC PRINCIPLES OF DEMENTIA CARE**

Instructor's Version with Answers for Handout 2-3

● REAL-LIFE SCENARIO

A Day in the Life of Pat

Pat is a client in the middle stages of AD. After mealtime, Pat frequently wanders into other clients' rooms causing the residents to become upset. Numerous times, staff had to physically remove Pat from the residents' rooms to be medicated. Pat has been restrained and monitored at the nurses' station to prevent wandering and maintain safety.

1. List the behaviors exhibited by Pat in this scenario. How would you classify the behaviors?
   - *Agitation*
   - *Combativeness*
   - *Repetitive behaviors*
   - *Wandering*
   - *Uncooperative behavior*
   - *Delusions*
   - *Catastrophic reactions*

   Pat's behaviors are challenging behaviors. Challenging behaviors are those that can lead to more troublesome events if not interceded. Interventions should be swift to avoid further problems. Without interventions from the staff, the behaviors can become harmful. Harmful behaviors have the potential to cause injury to the client or others.

2. What questions should the staff be exploring to develop potential solutions?
   - *Find the who, what, where, when, and why of the behavior.*
   - *Does the client need or want something?*
   - *Is there something in the environment causing the behavior?*
   - *How is the staff responding to the behavior?*

3. What intervention from the staff, in the scenario, should be avoided whenever possible?

   Medicating and restraining should be the last resort for controlling challenging behaviors. To better support clients and those around them, the staff should intervene at the first sign of frustration and avoid a combative episode. Staff should use a calming voice and redirect the client from wandering by introducing a simple task. For example, "Pat, will you bring me the trays." Or they can evoke a conversation: "Tell me about your pet."

   After defusing the potential problem, the staff should observe and report any indications for the wandering and modify the environment to discourage the behavior. For instance, does the wandering occur when Pat does not finish all the food, after playing bingo, or when family visits. The client may not like the meal served and could be looking for additional food. The client may be fatigued after the morning activity and wants to rest. Pat may be looking for loved ones. Any potential causes and solutions should be incorporated into the client's plan of care and communicated to all appropriate staff.

GROUP ACTIVITY

The purpose of this activity is to reinforce how outside influences can affect mood, performance, and behaviors. The following activity can be completed as a class, in small groups, or individually.

Explore how the following situations affect your mood, performance, and behavior. Discuss your answers.

- Being hungry.
- Not knowing anyone when entering an event or party.
- Feeling cold.
- Being lost on a highway or in a strange city.
- Running late for an appointment or picking up your child.
- Being held against your will.
- Having a headache.
- Being locked out of your home or car.
- Not knowing the answers on a test.
- Waking up in a strange place.
- Trying to speak and understand a foreign language.

Name _____ Date _____

Program/Course _____ Instructor's Name _____

Basic Principles of Care Pre- and Post-Test

1. What is the most important aspect of caring for a client with dementia?
   a. Safety
   b. Routines
   c. Communication
   d. All of the above

2. A client with dementia is requesting to see her deceased mother. What should the caregiver do?
   a. Reorient the client to time and place and tell her that her mother is dead.
   b. Validate the client's feelings and ask the client to share something about her mother.
   c. Confirm that the client is talking about her mother and not confusing her with the client's daughter.
   d. Use therapeutic touch and then move on to a more coherent client requiring help.

3. The communication process involves perception, evaluation, and transmission of information. What part of the process is affected with dementia?
   a. The dementia client has a problem with perception due to the damage to the temporal lobes of the brain.
   b. The dementia client has a problem with perception, evaluation, and transmission due to the damage to the temporal lobes of the brain.
   c. The dementia client has a problem with evaluation due to the damage to the occipital lobe of the brain.
   d. The dementia client has a problem with perception, evaluation, and transmission due to the damage to the occipital lobe of the brain.

4. When a dementia client is uncooperative about brushing his teeth, how should the caregiver first respond?
   a. The caregiver should ask the nurse to increase the client's prescription medications.
   b. The caregiver should distract the client and introduce a new activity and then try the activity again when the client is calmer.
   c. The caregiver should instruct the family to ask for a physical exam to rule out a medical cause for the behavioral change.
   d. The caregiver should ignore the change so as not to reinforce the negative behavior.

(continued)

Handout **2-1**

Basic Principles of Care Pre- and Post-Test
(Continued)

5. What is a catastrophic reaction?
   a. A catastrophic reaction is a method of assessing and recording eye movements by measuring the electric activity of the extraocular muscles.
   b. A catastrophic reaction is a common side effect from most antianxiety medications.
   c. A catastrophic reaction is a brief interruption of brain function, usually lasting a few seconds.
   d. A catastrophic reaction is an extreme emotional response to a trivial event, leading to sudden mood changes, crying, screaming, or even physical violence.

Basic Principles of Dementia Care

- Use effective communication skills.

- Reduce distractions and avoid information overload.

- Positively address feelings of insecurity.

- Use message boards, signs, or pictures.

- Use touch.

- Pick "your" battles.

- Do not take the behaviors personally.

- Center "yourself."

A Day in the Life of Pat: A Real-Life Scenario

Pat is a client in the middle stages of AD. After mealtime, Pat frequently wanders into other clients' rooms, causing the residents to become upset. Numerous times, staff had to physically remove Pat from the residents' rooms to be medicated. Pat has been restrained and monitored at the nurses' station to prevent wandering and maintain safety.

1. List the behaviors exhibited by Pat in this scenario. How would you classify the behaviors?

2. What questions should the staff be exploring to develop potential solutions?

3. What intervention from the staff, in the scenario, should be avoided whenever possible?

Handout **2-3**

MODULE 2 BASIC PRINCIPLES OF DEMENTIA CARE

Developing a Plan of Care

- **Maintain physical health**
- **Maintain a supportive physical environment**
- **Maintain a supportive social environment**

Behavioral and Memory Interventions

- **Task breakdown technique**
- **Montessori-based activities**
- **Space-retrieval practice**
- **Validation therapy**

The Communication Process

- Perception
- Evaluation
- Transmission

Common Communication Characteristics with AD

- **Verbal stereotypic language**
- **Empty speech**
- **Paraphasias**
- **Rules of conversation omitted**
- **Windows of lucidity**

Conversational Techniques

- Observe non-verbal communication
- Maintain a calming approach
- Approach the client from the front
- Use therapeutic touch
- Use questions that offer choices

Conversational Techniques (*cont.*)

- **Stimulate conversations**
- **Assist with word searching**
- **Avoid giving orders**
- **Allow time for a response**

Causes for Behavioral Changes

- **Physical discomfort**
- **Lack of recognition**
- **Over stimulation**
- **Difficulty completing tasks/activities**
- **Inability to communicate effectively**

Exploring Causes and Solutions to Behavioral Changes

- **Determine the type of behavior**
- **Identify the behavior**
- **Explore potential solutions**
- **Seek alternative approaches**

Common Behavioral Symptoms

- **Apathy**
- **Anxiety**
- **Agitation**
- **Combativeness**

Common Behavioral Symptoms (*cont.*)

- **Repetitive behaviors**
- **Hoarding**
- **Wandering**
- **Sleep disturbances**

Common Behavioral Symptoms (cont.)

- Sexual behavior
- Uncooperative behaviors
- Accusations/suspiciousness/paranoia
- Delusions
- Catastrophic reaction

Module 3
Daily Care

Goal
To understand how to assist with the daily care needs of the dementia client.

Objectives
After completion of the presentation, students will be able to:
- Describe the plan of care regarding daily care needs.
- Describe the task breakdown technique for bathing.
- Describe the basic principles of care when assisting with bathing.
- List possible causes of dressing difficulties.
- Describe the basic principles of care when assisting with oral care.
- List five ways cognitive changes interfere with toileting.
- Define a toileting regime.

GENERAL INFORMATION/OVERVIEW

Lecture Material for Slide 3-1

AD is a progressive, degenerative disease that affects the neurons of the brain, causing them to die at an abnormally increased rate. As the disease devours the brain cells, the AD clients are no longer able to process their surroundings. They frequently show impairments in their reasoning, judgment, and understanding. Dementia usually impacts the activities of daily living.

The client needs to use other functioning portions of the brain to complete tasks.

- As the population ages it is becoming more and more important to learn about dementia and AD.
- To be able to care for AD and dementia clients successfully, caregivers need to have a deeper understanding of their needs and their world.
- The burdens of daily care are commonly the reason for admission to long-term care facilities.
- As clients deteriorate, their unwillingness to dress and bathe themselves becomes troublesome for the caregiver

DAILY CARE

Lecture Material for Slide 3-2

Daily care is inclusive of mealtime, recreation, personal care, and ambulation. This module focuses on personal care. The activities are all private and personal, and clients have performed them independently for most of their lives. Alteration in cognition leads clients to be unaware of their disabilities. Caregivers and clients are now faced with the reality of their limitations.

- When caring for a cardiac or orthopedic client, for example, interventions are basic and routine. Conversely, the interventions needed for the dementia client are far from ordinary. The process needs to be adapted frequently to the ever changing behaviors associated with dementia.
- Short-term memory loss is the result of damage in the hippocampus. As a result of the memory loss, the caregiver must incorporate the frequent and repetitious redirection of instructions.
- The AD client cannot be rushed or hurried. The decrease in brain synapses inhibits the ability to multitask. The client is unable to integrate the steps. The caregiver's sense of urgency can be transferred to the client, leading to behavioral changes. Even when the caregiver is experiencing time restraints, speak calmly, slowly, and modify the plan of care. (See Module 2 for lecture material regarding behavioral changes.)
- In the past, when clients entered a care facility with the diagnosis of AD, they were medicated to remain calm and left to wither away. No longer is this an acceptable practice. With the person-centered approach, interventions are client specific and designed to extend their independence.

- A recent study showed increases in the longevity of mental skills with early-stage AD clients when given mental stimulation exercises. The AD client now can live a meaningful life with the proper care and understanding.
- Incorporate all aspects of daily care as part of an activity. No longer should bathing be a task. The bathing process creates a relationship between the caregiver and the client.

Plan of Care

- Developing a plan of care consists of incorporating the client's physical health, and maintaining a supportive physical, and social environment.
- The priorities of care and the strategies to achieve the goals are defined.
- After each activity is completed, the caregiver evaluates the extent to which the goals of care have been achieved.
- Modifications are made when necessary to accommodate the client's deteriorating abilities.
- The plan of care for the client with dementia is constantly modified due to the nature of the disease.

MAINTAINING PHYSICAL HEALTH

Lecture Material for Slide 3-3

Every client requires a full-body assessment. Observe all aspects of the client to determine his or her capabilities.

- Assess how the client interacts with the environment.
- Observing the client during all aspects of daily care provides important assessment information. Use all the senses when observing the client (touch, sight, smell, hearing, taste).
- Detect weaknesses and how the weaknesses affect the client's ability to perform ADL.
- By detecting the smallest changes, the caregiver can adapt interventions to the client's strengths.
- Observe and determine the client's communication abilities. The process of communication includes perception, evaluation, and transmission. The spoken word must be heard, comprehended, and then implemented.
- By speaking with AD clients, the caregiver can determine their needs and wants, while encouraging conversation. Utilizing dialogue stimulates the frontal lobe area of the brain, where the speech center is located. The continual stimulation of the brain may help the client retain adequate communication skills.
- Remember to listen to clients through verbal and nonverbal communication. Maintain eye contact and acknowledge their

conversation. Be aware of facial expressions and body language; expressions can be very telling of thoughts. Gesture during conversations to confirm interest. The importance of listening cannot be stressed enough.

- Use the client's feedback as much as possible to maintain autonomy and self-esteem. Create an environment that allows freedom and structure.

Identifying the Client's Strengths and Weaknesses

Observe the client for:

- Stamina level for the independent completion of daily care.
- Physical limitations resulting from comorbid conditions.
- Memory recall of the layout of the facility.
- Cognitive abilities to determine the steps of bathing, dressing, oral care, and toileting.
- Attention levels to initiate, maintain, and terminate the activity.
- Visuospatial adaptation for completion of the task.
- Coordination of movement to complete bathing, dressing, oral care, and toileting.
- Language skills for the articulation of needs.
- Judgment to assure safety.

MAINTAINING THE PHYSICAL ENVIRONMENT

Lecture Material for Slide 3-4

AD clients require the continued monitoring of their physical environment. Due to the alteration in cognition, their abilities are ever changing. A structured environment is necessary to compensate for cognitive loss.

- Client routines need to stay constant to help create a secure environment.
- Using a person-centered approach helps determine clients' pre-illness routines. For example, did they bathe in the morning or the evening? Did they prefer baths or showers? Did they wear dresses or pants? Did they wear makeup? Implementing their routines utilizes their preserved or procedural memory process, reinforcing their involvement in self-care.
- All interventions are person-centered, reflect client capabilities, and emphasize flexibility. The AD client may successfully perform a task one day and not the next. The deterioration of the neurons resembles a faulty appliance wire, working randomly. Routine interventions need to be adapted accordingly to achieve a successful activity.
- Minimize the client's fears and anxieties. No matter how well clients appear; the disease is always impacting their environment.
- AD clients can lose 30% of their brain cell function before any deterioration is seen. They may appear cognitively intact, but in fact

they need redirection and help with certain tasks. As the disease progresses, they need to be redirected and coached with every step of the process.

Providing a Safe Environment

- Adapt the environment to accommodate physical disabilities.
- Utilize the required adaptive devices to encourage independence.
- Create memory aids as a reminder.
- Maintain clutter-free walkways and pathways.
- Avoid wet floor areas.
- Maintain well lit areas.
- Use stairs cautiously, avoiding them when possible.
- Store medications or other hazardous items out of the client's reach.

Lecture Material for Slide 3-5

MAINTAINING A SUPPORTIVE SOCIAL ENVIRONMENT

Too often when people hear someone has been diagnosed with dementia, the client is ignored and not included in decision making. Always encourage participation.

- Treat clients as adults, no matter what their cognitive level. The brain retains and processes emotions in a different way than factual memories. Social skills usually remain intact longer than decision making and intuition.
- Remember not to impose personal values on the client, such as how often they need to bathe, change clothes, or shave.
- Encourage clients to perform tasks that highlight their strengths. Circumvent their weaknesses by developing alternate solutions. Participation in activities provides the opportunity for relationships with others and fulfills most psychosocial needs.
- Praise all attempted appropriate activities. Use positive redirection without focusing on the failed segment of the task. If clients are on their way to the bathroom and become distracted, redirect them with the use of a word or phrase, "Let's go to the bathroom." A common response from the client may be, "I was on my way there, wasn't I?"
- Incorporate the individual's interests and hobbies into the caregiver-client relationship. Look for activities the client is still able to perform and focus on them. Use previous habits as a purposeful activity. Consider the client's previous grooming habits. For example, a woman who used to wear makeup can still wear lipstick.
- Encourage all successful activities to promote self-esteem and usefulness.
- The temporal lobe of the brain is responsible for understanding the spoken word. The cognitive deficit prevents normal nerve

transmission, resulting in lost data. Challenging behaviors occur when the client's expected result does not materialize. For example, "Let's get washed, then we'll have breakfast." The client may retain only the last portion of the statement, becoming agitated when led to the bathroom. Explain one idea at a time.

- The disease process evokes confusion. The deterioration in the brain cell pathways in the amygdala and hippocampus often leads to anger and frustrations. Displaced anger is not to be taken personally; the client's reactions are part of the disease process.

- During daily care, furnish an environment that provides clients with adequate privacy. Though their cognitive abilities are failing, their sense of pride and dignity remain. Providing privacy in the bathroom creates a more desirable atmosphere for them, thus reducing incontinence. Incontinence and refusal to bathe may be directly related to a lost sense of privacy.

Options: Competency for bathing can be reviewed during this portion of lecture.

Lecture Material for Slides 3-6 and 3-7

Slide 3-6

BATHING

Bathing an AD client poses numerous obstacles. Clients with dementia may pay less attention to personal hygiene.

Causes of Bathing Difficulties

- With their social judgment and awareness diminished, AD clients' loss of independence is threatened, by becoming dependent on others for bathing and grooming.

- All aspects of the bathing process become muddled for the AD client: adjusting the water temperature, maneuvering in and out of the shower, and the use of a washcloth.

- The short-term memory deterioration requires continual redirection. The client may forget the reason for the bath, the bathing sequence, and/or its supplies.

- The fact of being nude and feeling closed in may trigger anxiety and vulnerability.

- Too much stimulation can cause the client to become agitated and refuse to continue the bathing process altogether.

- Personalize the plan of care to the client's needs. To reduce conflict over bathing, try either substituting a sponge or towel bath or reducing the frequency of bathing.

- Encourage the use of an electric razor to promote independence with shaving. Remind the client to shave. If the client customarily used a traditional razor, replace it with a safety razor and supervise the activity.

- Persons with dementia may forget about, or have difficulty with, cutting their nails. Maintain appropriate grooming to the fingernails and toenails. Remember to file nails only as needed and not to cut. Refer the client to the facility podiatrist if toenails need to be cut.
- Allow clients to perform as much of a given task independently as possible. For example, if they are unable to style their own hair, have them brush their own hair and then assist with styling.

Slide 3-7

Suggested interventions

- Prior to the clients' bathing, gather all the required supplies and prepare the workspace. Organization eliminates undue stress. Clients excel in a calm and relaxed environment.
- To avoid startling the client, approach from the front. Their altered depth perception and peripheral vision is the result of occipital lobe damage.
- Speak calmly; their emotions are unbalanced and a harsh voice can be frightening.
- Use a gentle touch to calm and reassure clients.
- Announce bath time immediately prior to the activity.
- Limit choices to reduce decision-making anxiety.
- Set the bathroom at a comfortable temperature. Set the water temperature for clients if necessary. (They may be unable to gauge the water temperature.)
- Provide privacy by closing the door and having a robe available.
- Observe and report any physical changes in the client (skin breakdown, shortness of breath, or pain).
- Use task-breakdown technique. State each step of the process separately. Give only one command at a time. For example, "Take the washcloth." "Here is the soap." Reassure clients throughout the task.
- Involve and coach the client in the bathing process.
- Never leave clients alone while bathing. They may appear competent, while in reality their judgment is impaired.
- Dry the client's skin completely, paying special attention to the skin folds.
- Distract the anxious client with redirection. Be flexible.
- Encourage conversation when appropriate.
- Reinforce and praise all positive behaviors.
- Report all changes in behavior and routine to the supervisor.

Things to Know

- Schedule the bath at the same time of the day.
- If the client persistently refuses to bathe, try again after he or she has rested.

- Clients may become agitated by a reflection in the mirror. Changes in the brain create visual and recognition loss. They may not recognize their reflection or may believe there are strangers in the room. Covering or removing mirrors may be appropriate.
- The sensation of cascading water on their face may be disturbing to the client. Utilizing a washcloth may minimize anxiety. Separate hair washing from bathing for the same reason.
- When taking a bath, fill the tub with only a few inches of water. With the loss of depth perception and recognition, clients may interpret the bath water as a danger.
- Provide a safe environment. Check for throw rugs or loose carpeting in the bathroom. Reinforce the use of handrails to prevent falls in the shower. A skid-proof tub mat minimizes falls in the shower.
- Avoid the use of bubble bath or bath oil. The mixture creates a slippery surface.
- Use liquid soap rather than bar soap.

Audience Interaction for Slides 3-6 and 3-7

Ask the audience how they would respond to a client who was refusing to bathe. Remember to include the client's interpretation of the event. Review the following in the discussion:

- Maintain a bathing routine.
- Use distraction.
- Gently guide the client to the bath area.
- Modify the plan of care.
- Use a person-centered approach.
- Discuss fears, including those from the pre-illness state.

Lecture Material for Slides 3-8 and 3-9

Slide 3-8

ORAL CARE

Oral care is the most likely activity to be neglected when someone is unable to perform self-care. Inadequate oral care can result in serious medical problems with the teeth and gums, or possibly create systemic infections.

Causes of Oral Care Difficulties

- Lack of judgment, poor coordination, and altered depth perception make performing oral care challenging. The client may not understand what dental care is or its importance.
- Proper oral hygiene involves the cleanliness, comfort, and moisturizing of mouth structures.
- Simple swabbing of the mouth is ineffective in removing food debris.
- Oral care should be performed a least twice daily, in the morning and prior to bedtime. Choose the time of day the client is most calm. If the client begins to resist, stop, distract, and try again.
- Periodic exams by a dentist should continue as long as possible.

- A daily inspection of the oral cavity is recommended to ensure that no inflammation, swelling, or tenderness is occurring. The client may not be able to express discomfort.
- Tensed facial expression, facial rubbing, or the refusal to eat during mealtime may be a signal of alterations in the oral cavity.

Altered mucous membranes can be related to:
- Dehydration.
- Ineffective hygiene.
- Mediations.
- Ill fitting dentures.
- Endotracheal intubation.

Causes of oral cavity pain:
- Loose teeth are the result of poor nutrition, hygiene and medications.
- Gingivitis is a condition in which the gums are red, swollen, and bleed. Poor oral hygiene, diabetes mellitus, leukemia, or vitamin deficiency are causes of gingivitis.
- Glossitis is an inflammation of the tongue resulting from an infectious disease, burn, bite, or other injury.

Oral care is vital to everyone, even those with no natural teeth (endentulous). The gums and oral tissues need to be cleaned and massaged daily.

Procedure for Assisting with Oral and Denture Care

- Use simple commands to guide the client throughout each portion of the task.
- Check the client's mouth, including the insides of the cheeks, for signs of gum inflammation, swelling, or tenderness.
- Assess the client's abilities to determine the level of assistance required.

Instruct the client to:
- Brush all surfaces in the mouth to remove food particles and plaque.
- Brush the inner and outer surfaces of the upper and lower teeth by brushing from the gum to the crown of each tooth.
- Use short strokes, brushing one tooth at a time. Continue until the entire mouth is completed.
- Floss the teeth. Use flossing devices if the client is unable to maneuver dental floss.
- Rinse the mouth thoroughly. Repeat rinsing as necessary.

Instruct the client with dentures to:
- Remove dentures. Use store-bought denture cleaners as directed.
- Use short strokes to clean the denture plate.
- Clean the soft tissues of the mouth at least once daily.

- Use a soft toothbrush, sponge, or washcloth wrapped around the finger to brush the gums.
- Include brushing the gum line to stimulate circulation and to remove additional food particles.
- Rinse the mouth thoroughly. Repeat rinsing as necessary.

Slide 3-9 | Suggested Interventions

- Prior to oral care, gather all required supplies and prepare the workspace.
- Approach the client from the front.
- Speak calmly.
- Use a gentle touch to calm and reassure the client.
- Announce the task immediately prior to the activity.
- Limit choices to reduce decision-making anxiety.
- Use the task-breakdown technique.
- Ensure privacy.
- Provide a comfortable and safe work area for the client.
- Encourage participation. Have the client hold the toothbrush when applying the toothpaste.
- Reinforce and praise all positive behaviors.
- Encourage conversation when appropriate.
- Distract the anxious client with redirection. Be flexible.
- Report any changes in the client's condition.

Oral Care for an Unconscious Client

Providing mouth care for an unconscious individual requires keeping the mouth moist and eliminating secretions. If the client is unable to eat or drink, or is a mouth breather, the mucosa tends to dry and crust may form on the tongue and mucous membranes.

Suggested Interventions for the Unconscious Client

- Explain the procedure to the client even if confused or unresponsive.
- Wash hands.
- Assemble supplies.
- Provide privacy.
- Position the client and then turn the client's head toward the caregiver.
- Place a towel under the client's face and the emesis basin under the client's chin.
- Carefully separate the upper and lower teeth with the padded tongue blade.

- Clean the mouth using the toothettes or tongue blade moistened with mouthwash or water.
- Suction as needed.
- Clean the crown and inner surfaces first.
- Swab the roof of the mouth and inside cheeks and lips.
- Wash the tongue, avoiding the gag reflex.
- Moisten a clean applicator with water and swab the client's mouth to rinse.
- Repeat as needed.
- Apply ointment to lips.
- Explain to the client that the procedure is complete.
- Reposition the client.
- Clean the equipment and return it to the proper place.
- Wash hands.
- Report any changes in the client's condition.

Things to Know

- Establish and maintain a daily routine.
- Use mirroring by standing in front of the client and showing him or her the act of brushing.
- Inspect the client's mouth daily; observe for sensitivity, swelling, and sores.
- Use adaptive devices to aid in the tooth-brushing process, such as elongated toothbrushes, and suctioning toothbrushes.
- Use ingestible toothpaste for clients who tend to swallow the toothpaste.
- If the client becomes uncooperative and clenches the lips and cheeks together, use a toothbrush bent backward at 45 degrees. (To bend the toothbrush, run it under hot water.) Slide the bent brush into the corner of the mouth to break the muscle spasms and help lift the cheek out of the way.
- Be flexible.
- Modify oral care when faced with resistance. Use denture foam applicators, for example.

Things to Know about Dentures

- Clients with dentures must be reminded to clean their dentures daily and assisted in doing so. As their condition declines, additional support will be needed.
- Clients eat better with properly fitting dentures. Poorly fitting dentures can lead to mouth sores, irritation, dehydration, and constipation.

Audience Interaction for Slides 3-8 and 3-9

- When a client loses weight, their dentures may not fit properly. Monitor the client's weight to ensure proper nutrition and properly fitting dentures.

Ask the audience to share oral care techniques that have been successfully applied to clients.

Lecture Material for Slide 3-10

DRESSING

Inappropriate dressing can be one of the problems faced by family members when caring for a client with dementia.

Causes of Dressing Difficulties

- The client can no longer coordinate outfits, may put undergarments on last, or fasten buttons in the wrong order.
- The individual may lack the necessary decision-making skills required to select the appropriate attire for the weather.
- The client may be unaware of the passing of time and resist daily clothing changes. Do not argue when the client insists on wearing the same outfit every day.
- In the early stages of the disease, simplify the client's clothing options. Use coordinating colors for easy matching. Use labeling to help the client locate clothing articles in his or her room.
- Limit clothing choice, but encourage participation. Ask the client, "Do you want to wear the pink shirt or the yellow one?" The option heard last is usually the preference. Posing the question offers the client a purposeful event and stimulates conversation.
- Lay out the clothing in the order of the dressing sequence. (Undergarments should be the top layer in the layout.) By decreasing the client's risk for error, the activity is successful, thus enhancing self-esteem.
- Eliminate clutter and distraction while the client is dressing.
- Reduce the amount of accessories worn. The additional items may become burdensome. Maintain the client's personality, but use simpler garments to mimic the familiar look. If the client routinely wore scarves, for example, use those that have Velcro® for easy fastening. The client's safety comes before fashion. Be mindful of possible dangers.
- As the disease progresses, there may be noticeable stiffening of the muscles. Choose clothing that maintains the client's independence in dressing (avoid small buttons, hooks, and other hard-to-handle features).

Lecture Material for Slide 3-11

Causes of Undressing in Public

Clothing choices should be appropriate for the temperature in the room and comfortable. When dementia clients become overheated, they may undress in public areas. The same is true if the garments are uncomfortable. Find the who, what, where, and why for the public undressing.

- Is the client too warm?
- Does the client need to use the bathroom?
- Is the client fatigued and preparing for bed?
- Is the client bored?

Suggested interventions

- Gather all the required supplies and prepare the workspace.
- Provide privacy.
- Approach the client from the front.
- Speak calmly.
- Use a gentle touch to calm and reassure the client.
- Announce the task immediately prior to the activity.
- Limit clothing choices.
- Set the room at a comfortable temperature.
- Use the task-breakdown technique.
- Hand the client the clothes while giving the instruction.
- Encourage the client to perform as much of the task independently as possible.

Things to Know about Clothing Suggestions

- Use clothes that are easy to put on and take off.
- Busy prints can be distracting to the client, use simple patterned fabric.
- Avoid placing irritating materials, like wool or rough synthetic fabrics, against the skin.
- Use undergarments or T-shirts that are comfortable if put on backward or forward.
- Eliminate the use of bras if troublesome for the female client. If a bra is necessary, have the woman lean forward, place the bra over the breasts, pull it to support, and snap.
- Avoid buttons, zippers, or snaps.
- Use Velcro® for clothes and shoes.
- The clothes should be loose and nonrestrictive.
- Elastic waistbands make for comfort and ease for toileting.
- Make sure the clothing length is appropriate for the client to prevent falls.

- Buy several outfits of the same color, including socks. The uniformity helps with familiarity and limits choices.
- Shoes should provide support and have a rubber sole. Avoid laces.
- Compliment clients on their appearance.
- Continue any pre-illness style, unless potentially restrictive or dangerous (pants, suits, dresses, jewelry).

Audience Interaction for Slide 3-11

Ask the audience to share any helpful strategies when assisting a client with dressing.

Lecture Material for Slide 3-12

TOILETING

Toileting is a complex occurrence with many phases that may be unpleasant for caregivers and clients with AD. Providing physical and cognitive support can calm the emotionally distraught AD client and avoid catastrophic reactions.

- As the AD progresses, clients may begin to experience bowel and bladder disturbances.
- Incontinence may result due to the decline of intellect and memory.
- Clients may no longer recognize the feelings of elimination (pressure and urgency). They may no longer distinguish between the signal to void and a bowel movement. They may not remember how, when, and where to respond to toileting needs.

Decreased cognitive abilities interfere with:
- Comprehending the urge to toilet.
- Holding the urine or stool until it is appropriate to go to the bathroom.
- Locating the bathroom.
- Recognizing the commode.
- Using the toilet correctly.

Lecture Material for Slides 3-13 and 3-14

Slide 3-13

INCONTINENCE

Incontinence is the loss of control of bladder and/or bowel function. The elderly and especially people with dementia, have a higher incidence of urinary incontinence. Urinary incontinence is common with the elderly and is more prevalent with people with dementia. Males have an equal or greater frequency of incontinence than females.

- Measures can be incorporated into the daily routine to alleviate the problem of incontinence or lessen its burden.
- Incontinence can be very distressing for the person with dementia. Remain calm; use gentle words to help reduce the client's embarrassment.

- People with dementia, just like other adults, are susceptible to medical causes of incontinence. Many of these conditions are treatable under medical supervision.
- Bladder and bowel incontinence should be discussed with the client's physician to determine if an underlying medical problem exists. Notify the supervisor if the incidence of incontinence changes.
- In order to incorporate interventions for incontinence into the plan of care, the caregiver needs to monitor the client's toileting habits. By determining the cause and type of incontinence, client specific interventions can be incorporated into their daily routine. Always focus on the client's strengths and support any weaknesses. Once achieved, a toileting regime can be developed.

Reasons for Incontinence

- Incontinence with quick onset may be the result of a urinary tract infection, fecal impaction, or constipation.
- In the early stages of the disease, clients may deny the incontinence to reduce embarrassment. They may try to hide the soiled clothes. The realization of the impairment may be too upsetting for them to accept.
- In the later stages of the illness, the incontinence results from the reduction in the cerebral cortex neurons (nerve cells). With the decrease in the number of nerve cells, no impulses are sent from the micturition center (controls urination) of the brain to the bladder.
- As clients become more disoriented and unaware of their environment, they may void in inappropriate places.
- Clients should be monitored to determine the reason for their incontinence.

Observing the Client's Incontinent Behavior

- Is the client incontinent of urine, stool, or both?
- How often is the client incontinent?
- When is the client incontinent?
- When did the problem start?
- How soiled is the client? Saturated? Just a trickle?
- What was the client doing when the incontinence occurred?
- Has there been any change in the client's condition or environment?
- Has the client complained of any pain when toileting? Any fever?
- Have there been changes in the medication regime?
- Does the client pass urine in a strange place?

Slide 3-14

Medical Causes of Incontinence

- Infection (urinary tract infection)
- Constipation

- Medication
- Hormonal changes
- Enlarged prostate

Lecture Material for Slide 3-15

URINARY INCONTINENCE

Urinary incontinence is the inability to retain urine. The causes of the incontinence vary. Many forms are treatable while others are more difficult to manage. In either case the condition is embarrassing and may impact socialization. Finding the cause of the incontinence is essential to promoting self-esteem.

Types of Urinary Incontinence

- Stress incontinence
- Urge incontinence
- Overflow incontinence
- Functional incontinence

Stress Incontinence

- Stress incontinence is the result of a weak urinary sphincter and/or perineal muscles. The weakness allows small amounts of urine to pass when the intra-abdominal pressure is suddenly increased and surpasses the pressure of the internal sphincter.
- Frequently the incontinence occurs when the client stands up, coughs, or sneezes. The client is usually dry between occurrences.

Urge Incontinence

- Urge incontinence is the result of the inner muscular lining of the bladder not being strong enough to handle the pressure of the internal sphincter. (This is also known as spastic bladder, unstable bladder, or uninhibited bladder.)
- In late-stage AD the number of neurons in the micturition center have decreased. This causes the unwanted contraction of the bladder prior to being full.
- The client is usually continuously wet.

Overflow Incontinence

- Unlike other types of incontinence, overflow is the result of a blockage in the urethra. Males with benign prostatic hypertrophy (BPH) commonly experience overflow incontinence.
- When the pressure in the bladder exceeds the pressure of the sphincter, small amounts of urine are passed.
- The client usually has a larger than normal bladder, which can be felt upon palpation. The client usually never is able to completely empty the bladder resulting in frequent urinary tract infection.

Functional Incontinence

- Functional incontinence occurs when clients are aware they need to void and just cannot get to the bathroom in time.
- Commonly, stress incontinence preempts functional incontinence.

Lecture Material for Slides 3-16 and 3-17

Slide 3-16

TOILETING REGIMEN

Toileting programs and drug treatments can help the management of urinary incontinence with clients with dementia.

- Prompted toileting regimes have been shown to reduce incontinence by an average of 32% and appear to be a useful approach in managing incontinence.
- Clients who are severely cognitively impaired, are the least mobile, and have the greatest frequency of incontinence, derive the least benefit from toileting programs. Palliative measures may be more appropriate in these cases.
- Determine the client's strengths and weaknesses for toileting to develop a toileting regime. Evaluate the plan of care and modify it as needed.
- Since clients' cognitive abilities may appear intact, closely monitor their skill level. Do not assume they are going to the bathroom just because they were reminded.
- Observe the client's toileting patterns. Suggest the use of the bathroom at regular intervals, incorporating it into their schedule.
- Create a daily routine. Remind the client to use the bathroom every two hours. The routine promotes the client's ability to retain the skill as long as possible.
- Learn clients' nonverbal signals for having to void. Observing their need-for-toileting cues helps reduce accidents. (Does the client tug at the belt? Does the client touch the genitals? Does the client utilize nonverbal sounds?)

Slide 3-17

- Use words that are familiar to the person, such as "pee" or "tinkle." If English is not their first language, use words in their native language.
- Place a sign on the bathroom door with a picture of a toilet. Leave the door open for clients who are unable to open doors. Use signs to remind clients to use toilet paper, flush the toilet, and wash their hands.
- The toilet should be comfortable for the client so they remain seated long enough for a bowel movement. Clients should be able to reach the floor and rest their feet comfortably.
- Place colored tape showing a pathway to the bathroom if the client frequently gets lost.

- The pathway to the bathroom and the bathroom itself should be well lit. Use a night-light to guide the client to the bathroom in the nighttime hours.
- If the client has trouble voiding, help him or her relax with music or the sound of running water.
- If the client has frequent accidents, do not chastise; provide positive reinforcement.

Determine the Client's Strengths and Weaknesses for Toileting

- What can the client do?
- What does the client do?
- How does he or she do it?
- Which parts of the task is the client unable to do?
- Why is he or she unable to do them?
- Where does he or she perform best?
- When does he or she perform best?

Suggested Interventions

- Assist the client with any necessary steps. Use the task-breakdown technique.
- Ensure the client's underwear is changed as needed to keep him or her clean and dry. If incontinence is a problem, make sure clients are washed carefully with warm water and dried thoroughly before putting on clean clothes. The skin must remain clean and dry to avoid skin breakdown.
- Maintain the client's toileting regime. Try toileting before and after meals and before bed.
- Do not rush the client.
- Make sure the toilet paper is accessible and in view.
- Maintain a safe environment (avoid wet floors, throw rugs, and similar hazards).
- Make sure the bathroom is a comfortable temperature.
- A grab bar or other stable objects can be used for stability. Use a raised toilet seat if appropriate.
- Report any changes in bowel and bladder habits to the supervisor. Observe for urine and stool odor, color and consistency.

Things to Know

- Encourage the client to drink adequate fluids. Many people with dementia forget to drink or no longer recognize the sensation of thirst. Proper hydration reduces the risk of a urinary tract infection.

- Reduce the client's caffeine intake. Caffeine is a bladder irritant and increases incontinence.
- Provide a high-fiber diet to prevent constipation and promote regularity. Encourage regular exercise.
- To reduce nighttime accidents, avoid fluids after dinner.
- Use simple clothing to make toileting easier (Velcro® elastic waistbands or other fasteners).
- Avoid white plastic toilet seats. Use contrasting colors for easier identification. Colored toilet water may assist the male client with aim when urinating.
- The AD client may accidentally throw items down the toilet. Place a safety lock on the toilet lid.
- AD clients frequently lock themselves in the bathroom; they cannot remember how to unlock the door and become trapped. Remove the locks on the bathroom doors and replace them with regular door handles.
- For those who are restless or hyperactive and will not sit on the toilet, allow them to get up and down a few times. Music may have a calming effect. Try giving them something distracting while on the commode.
- Remove wastepaper baskets or other items that may resemble a commode.
- Encourage the use of a bedside commode when ambulation becomes more difficult.
- Diapers may be appropriate for the incontinent client. Discuss the use of diapers with the family and the health care team. Diapering should be used only when necessary.
- Use rubberized sheets for nighttime incontinence. Make sure the person's skin does not come into contact with any protective plastics, because contact causes skin breakdown.

SUMMING UP

Maintaining personal hygiene with the AD client is troublesome. Altered cognition creates obstacles for the caregiver. Care for the AD client utilizes a person-centered approach, in which the interventions are client specific and intended to extend independence. The heath care professional develops a plan of care that includes the client's physical health, physical environment and social environment. The caregiver must include the person-centered approach when completing all aspects of ADL. Dealing with incontinence is a common aspect of AD care. Determine the cause of the problem and develop a person-centered plan of care to maintain self-esteem, health, and independence.

Instructor's Version with Answers for Handout 3-2

● REAL-LIFE SCENARIO
A Day in the Life of Pat

Pat is starting to forget the way to the bathroom. All the toiletries for the ADL are located in the bathroom down the hall. Pat is sometimes found roaming the hallway confused and needing redirection. Recently Pat was seen trying to use the wastepaper basket as a toilet.

1. List interventions to assist Pat in finding the bathroom.
    a. Make a pathway from Pat's room to the bathroom using reflective tape.
    b. Place a picture of a toilet on the bathroom door.
    c. Keep the pathway to the bathroom clear of clutter.
    d. Use any assistive devices needed to make the trip to the bathroom easier and safer.

2. List ways to prevent incontinence.
    a. Develop and maintain a toileting schedule.
    b. Use the task-breakdown technique.
    c. Praise all attempts to void independently.
    d. Place a lid over all the wastepaper baskets.

3. What should be included when developing a plan of care?
    a. Determine the client's pre-illness routines.
    b. Develop a plan of care consisting of incorporating the client's physical health, physical environment, and social environment goals.
    c. Determine the priorities of care and strategies to achieve the goals.
    d. After each activity is completed, evaluate the extent to which the goals of care have been achieved.
    e. Modify where necessary to accommodate the client's deteriorating abilities.

GROUP ACTIVITY

The purpose of this activity is to examine ways to complete personal care activities with a client with dementia. The following activities can be completed as a class, in small groups, or individually.

Option 1

Each participant role-plays as a caregiver and as a client with dementia. Choose a personal care task and have the student caregiver assist the student dementia client with the task, utilizing the concepts learned in the module. Reverse roles with another task.

Option 2

During the task allow for a "difficult moment." Discuss solutions and alternative ways to handle the scenario.

Name _____ Date _____

Program/Course _____ Instructor's Name _____

Daily Care Pre- and Post-Test

1. What is the best time to schedule personal hygiene?
   a. Whenever is most convenient for the caregiver.
   b. At the same time of the pre-illness routine.
   c. When the client develops an odor.
   d. In the morning.

2. When assisting an AD client with a task:
   a. Be quick and to the point.
   b. Speak calmly.
   c. Give the client a time limit.
   d. Give them the instructions all at once.

3. What intervention is preferred with a dementia client who refuses to bathe?
   a. Yell and demoralize them.
   b. Use reality orientation and tell them they smell.
   c. Take their hand and force them into the shower.
   d. Move on to the next client and return at a later time.

4. Which is *not* a reason for providing proper oral care?
   a. Loose teeth, gingivitis, and halitosis
   b. Increases in caries (cavity) and ill fitting dentures
   c. Inability to eat, leading to weight loss
   d. Keeping the facility dentist busy

5. Which interventions can assist a dementia client with dressing?
   a. Providing privacy for the client
   b. Eliminating clutter and distraction when the client is dressing
   c. Laying out the clothing in the order of sequence for the client
   d. All of the above

Handout **3-1**

A Day in the Life of Pat: A Real-Life Scenario

Pat is starting to forget the way to the bathroom. All the toiletries for the ADL are located in the bathroom down the hall. Pat is sometimes found roaming the hallway confused and needing redirection. Recently Pat was seen trying to use the wastepaper basket as a toilet.

1. List interventions to assist Pat in finding the bathroom.

2. List ways to prevent incontinence.

3. What should be included when developing a plan of care?

Handout **3-2**

MODULE 3
DAILY CARE

Plan of Care

- **Incorporate goals**
- **Make goals attainable**
- **Re-evaluate**
- **Modify as needed**

Maintain Physical Health

- **Assess and observe**
- **Detect for strengths/ weaknesses**
- **Encourage communication**

Maintain Physical Environment

- **Maintain routines**
- **Use person-centered approach**
- **Maintain safety**

Maintain Social Environment

- **Treat as an adult**
- **Encourage activities**
- **Praise all attempted appropriate activities**
- **Incorporate previous habits**
- **Provide privacy**

Causes of Bathing Difficulties

- **Loss of independence**
- **Process becomes jumbled**
- **Privacy issues**
- **Forget the reason for bathing**

Bathing Interventions

- **Provide privacy/prepare work area**
- **Use task breakdown technique**
- **Promote independence**
- **Be flexible**
- **Observe and report changes**

Causes of Oral Care Difficulties

- **Lack of judgment**
- **Poor coordination**
- **Altered depth perception**
- **Forgetting the reason for oral care**

Oral Care

- **Prepare work space**
- **Use task breakdown technique**
- **Use mirroring**
- **Inspect the mouth daily**
- **Be flexible**
- **Observe and report changes**

Causes of Dressing Difficulties

- **Dressing sequences**
- **Clothing selections**
- **Unaware of passage of time**

Dressing

- **Limit clothing choices**
- **Use task breakdown technique**
- **Lay out clothing in dressing sequence**
- **Promote independence**
- **Continue pre-illness rituals**
- **Observe and report changes**

Toileting

Cognitive impairment interferes with:

- comprehending the urge to toilet
- the ability to hold urine/stool
- the ability to locate bathroom
- recognition of a commode
- the ability to use the toilet correctly

Incontinence/Toileting

- **Determine reasons for the incontinence**
- **Determine the type of incontinence**
- **Determine strengths and weaknesses**
- **Develop a toileting regime**

Medical Causes of Incontinence

- **Urinary tract infection**
- **Constipation**
- **Medication**
- **Hormonal changes**
- **Enlarged prostate**

Types of Urinary Incontinence

- **Stress**
- **Urge**
- **Overflow**
- **Functional**

Toileting Regimen

- **Prompt the client to toilet**
- **Determine strengths and weaknesses**
- **Observe patterns**
- **Create daily routine**
- **Learn verbal and non-verbal cues**

Toileting (cont.)

- Use familiar words ("pee")
- Use picture signs
- Place tape pathway to bathroom
- Create relaxing environment
- Do not chastise

Module 4
Eating Challenges with Dementia

Goal

To better understand the nutritional challenges of a client with dementia.

Objectives

After the completion of the presentation, students will be able to:

- List the components of a complete nutritional assessment.
- Describe how cognitive impairments can lead to eating challenges.
- Define ideational apraxia.
- Name four interventions that support the client's physical environment when eating.
- Describe the use of the Functional Abilities Assessment (FAA) tool.
- Describe the relationship between socialization and eating.
- Explain ways to prevent learned dependence.
- List at least four signs observed when a client has difficulty swallowing (dysphagia).

Lecture Material for Slide 4-1

GENERAL INFORMATION/OVERVIEW

As the debilitating disease of Alzheimer's progresses, clients become dependent in all their activities of daily living. Weight fluctuations are the greatest nutritional problem associated with Alzheimer's disease. Early on in the disease, depression may lead to anorexia. Restlessness may increase caloric demands or clients may simply forget to eat. Eating and swallowing are the last skills to be lost in the course of the illness. Prior to end-stage dementia, interventions can be implemented to prolong the ability to eat and provide successful, meaningful activities for the client and family.

- A person's food-related habits and preferences are based on cultural experiences and begin early in life. Social and moral values have been placed on eating. Food has been or can be used as a punishment or a reward.

- Eating is a highly social event. Studies demonstrate that people eat more when in a social environment.

- Emotions, social pressures, habits, taste, and the palatability of food all influence eating and drinking behaviors beyond the internal cues that control appetite.

- A recent study determined approximately 40% of Alzheimer's clients lose so much weight as the disease progresses that the loss threatens their general health. Physicians believe depression and loss of appetite may be the cause.

- Functional disabilities, gastrointestinal tract disorders, socioeconomic status, and social isolation can lead to a poor nutritional status.

- When more than 5% of normal body weight is unintentionally lost during a month, the implementation of a special dietary program is recommended.

- The elderly population over the age of 85, living independently, has been shown to have eating disabilities without a diagnosis of dementia. The rate of eating disabilities and eating dependence is higher in the nursing home population.

- The eating disabilities of clients living in long-term care facilities are related to: mobility impairment, cognitive impairment, upper extremity dysfunction, abnormal oral-motor function, the loss of teeth and dentures, abnormal swallowing, and mortality.

- Functional disabilities can prevent or alter the capacity of the elderly to obtain, prepare, and consume food. One study reported 39% of the elderly needed assistance with shopping, 26% needed help with meal preparation, and 6% needed help with eating.

- Eating is one of the last preserved abilities for the client with dementia. Theories suggest, because eating is the first activity of an infant and continues over the life span, it is fully integrated into the long-term memory.

Lecture Material for Slides 4-2 and 4-3

Slide 4-2

● PLAN OF CARE

Developing a plan of care consists of incorporating the client's physical health, physical environment, and social environmental goals. Eating behaviors can be improved by utilizing behavioral strategies. The nutritional goal for the client with dementia is to provide well-balanced meals and snacks. The plan should be person-centered, focusing on the client's likes, dislikes, and customs.

Maintaining Physical Health

Food and fluids are basic biological needs of all human beings. A nutritional assessment is an essential part of the plan of care. The assessment tool identifies clients who are at risk for dietary problems related to illness.

- A complete nutritional assessment includes observation, diagnostic testing dietary history, and anthropometric measures (body measurements).
- The screenings should also focus on current infections, the existence of pressure ulcers, or poor wound healing. Preventing any of these conditions is a priority.
- Special diets for comorbid conditions, such as diabetes and coronary artery disease, are incorporated into the plan.
- At the first appearance of eating problems, the client should be evaluated to rule out any acute medical conditions. Infections, stroke, pain, depression, anxiety, or side effects from medications can cause a reduction in food and fluid intake. Constipation is a frequent complaint in the elderly population and can cause anorexia.
- The client's swallowing ability should be carefully observed. A previous stroke may require changes in the texture of foods to accommodate difficulties with swallowing (dysphagia).
- Medications may create a dry mouth and throat, making eating or swallowing difficult.
- The condition of the oral cavity influences the ingestion of food. Mouth lesions, gum disease, loose teeth, or improperly fitting dentures affect a client's food intake. Fifty percent of Americans have lost all their teeth by age 65. Half of the nursing home population has problems with chewing, biting, and swallowing.
- Diet may have a significant impact on a drug's ability to work in the body. Prescription drugs and over-the-counter medicines contain ingredients that interact with the human body in different ways. Food and drug interactions can cause medications to become less effective or may lead to dangerous side effects. Various foods, beverages, alcohol, caffeine, and even cigarettes can interact with medications.
- The aging client often experiences decreased saliva production and gastric juices during the digestive process. These reductions lead to

difficulties with digestion and a larger number of food intolerances, resulting in heartburn and indigestion. The dementia client may be unable to communicate such symptoms, refuse to eat, or eat more to suppress the discomfort.

- The client's level of attention impacts food consumption. The ability to initiate, maintain, and terminate the act of eating is diminished with the alteration in attention. The individual may have difficulty staying seated at the table and does not finish a meal. The client may be drawn to a particular detail of the meal and disregard the remainder of the activity. For example, the client might pick up crumbs on the table instead of eating the food on the plate. The lack of initiative may prevent the client even from starting to eat.

Cognitive Impairments Leading to Eating Challenges

For individuals with cognitive impairments, mealtime can become a major undertaking. The social graces, table etiquette, and multiple tasks needed to prepare, serve, and eat a meal require higher brain functioning. Along with other activities, eating involves many complex tasks. When any of the cognitive functions are impaired, successful completion of a task is jeopardized. Memory loss and confusion alter the client's eating patterns. The memory loss may cause the client to forget to eat or to eat repetitively.

- Clients with dementia may no longer recognize the sensation of hunger and thirst.

- The brain can no longer process numerous thoughts simultaneously. Clients may become overwhelmed by the different foods on the plate and refuse to eat.

- The formation of tangles and plaques in the hypothalamus cause alterations in appetite and hunger. Clients may also lose their sense of smell and taste, reducing their desire to eat.

Slide 4-3

- Neuromuscular dyscoordination leaves clients with the inability to chew food, which creates difficulty with swallowing. Balance and position impairments may limit the client's ability to sit safely when eating. The client's decreased strength and endurance may contribute to poor dietary intake.

- Due to the damage in the parietal lobe, the client is unable to identify the purpose of objects. The table setting may look unfamiliar, leading clients to disregard the food items and utensils.

- Visual changes may influence nutritional intake. Clients may ignore objects in certain planes of vision. For example, the client may eat the food on only one side of the plate.

- The loss of communications skills limits the client's ability to request foods and fluids.

- Apraxia (the impaired ability to perform purposeful acts or to manipulate objects) leaves clients unable to use utensils or feed themselves.

IDEATIONAL APRAXIA

Lecture Material for Slides 4-4 and 4-5

Slide 4-4

Commonly, people diagnosed with dementia encounter problems feeding themselves due to ideational apraxia. Ideational apraxia is a specific type of apraxia that includes the loss of the ability to conceptualize, plan, prepare, and implement the intricate sequences of complex motor tasks involving objects, regardless of muscle sensation and coordination.

Eating Challenges of Persons with Ideational Apraxia:

- Not eating when the meal is placed in front of them
- Mixing foods together inappropriately
- Using the incorrect utensils when eating

Slide 4-5

- Attempting to eat foods still in the container or wrapper
- Eating inedible objects
- Incorrect sequencing of the eating task (eg, putting the fork in the mouth prior to placing food on it)

MAINTAINING A SUPPORTIVE PHYSICAL ENVIRONMENT

Lecture Material for Slides 4-6 and 4-7

Slide 4-6

Caring for the dementia client includes structuring the environment and activities in ways that compensate for cognitive loss. The client feels more secure when routines are established and maintained.

- Attempt to mimic the client's pre-illness routine. A regular routine enables the client to know what to expect. Change is acceptable when routines no longer work for the client. Clients in the early stages of their illness can adapt to modifications when appropriate.
- Consistency in the staff assignment benefits the client. Serve meals in an unrushed environment.
- Develop a fixed timetable or daily routine to include mealtimes and snacks.
- Provide a structured environment with identifiable cues for important destinations. Areas should have signs with illustrations to help clients gain orientation to their location. The dining hall and kitchen should be well designated.
- Limit extraneous noise and confusion in the surroundings. The cognitive deficits limit a person's ability to store simultaneous ideas.
- Dining rooms in nursing homes are often noisy. Clients are frequently seated long before meals are served. Excessive noise creates information overload, possibly triggering behavioral problems. Keep the noise level low and use music to mask other extrinsic sounds.

- A bright and cheery dining area is recommended. Brightness helps to eliminate dark corners and frightening shadows.

- Ensure the odor in the dining room is pleasant. A foul smelling room is unappetizing. Proper ventilation assists with comfort and scent.

- Seat the client in a relaxed position. Properly supportive chairs (eg, armchairs with back support) accommodate the client's limitations. Adapt the table height to the client's needs.

- The seating of clients should enhance the dining experience. Choose small dining rooms when appropriate to reduce distractions. Allow clients ample time to complete their meals. Incorporate extended mealtimes when suitable.

- Arrange for tablemates to be socially compatible. Integrate different functional levels to bring out clients' strengths.

Slide 4-7

- As the AD progresses, people frequently have problems with visual perception and discriminating objects from one another. The visual discrepancy makes it challenging for clients to distinguish a plate full of food from an ornate tablecloth or a white cup containing milk. Use contrasting colors to differentiate perimeters in the table setting.

- Research demonstrates that a brightly colored tablecloth with colorful plates and glasses promotes eating. The colorful tableware helps clients to see the food on their plates, leading to increased food consumption.

- Contrast the colors of the plates and the tablecloth. The alteration in vision prevents the client from identifying the difference between the plate and the tablecloth. Tablecloths also reduce reflective glare from tabletop surfaces.

- Adjust the eating environment to compensate for the client's physical limitations. Use modified plates and utensils.

- As the disease progresses, clients may forget the reason for the utensils. The use of finger foods prolongs clients' independence. Cutting foods into small finger-food sizes may be an option.

- Place only one selection of food on the plate at a time. Multiple choices are overwhelming and create agitation; clients may play with the food if they are unable to make a choice. Add additional food on the plate as it is consumed.

- Incorporate a variety of foods to ensure a healthy diet. Offer foods in several small meals during the day. Clients are more likely to consume more food with multiple seatings.

- Food jags may occur with dementia. Be flexible. Clients may like one food this week and dislike it next week.

- Use cues and prompts to reinforce eating. Encouraging clients to feed themselves helps with their dignity and self-esteem.

● MAINTAINING A SUPPORTIVE SOCIAL ENVIRONMENT

Lecture Material for Slide 4-8

Mealtime provides a perfect venue for conversation and interaction with staff and other residents. The social aspect of eating enhances the relationships with others, fulfilling the psychosocial need.

- Clients' attempts to communicate deserve positive acknowledgment. Encourage all attempts to socialize. Caregivers who respond to clients' efforts in a positive manner protect them from feelings of worthlessness and despair by fulfilling their basic needs.

- Remember basic conversational techniques. Maintain a calm and pleasant approach. Any personal emotions need to be neutralized before speaking with clients; be nonjudgmental. Caregivers can create successful meal intake when realizing the impact of their attitudes and actions on clients. The person with dementia mirrors surrounding moods.

- Most holidays and gatherings are centered on food. Eating has a complex social and emotional relationship. Gathering around a table during mealtime offers a sense of being included and connecting with others.

- Mealtime provides both the nourishment needed to survive and the socialization needed for positive self-esteem. Surrounding the client with a supportive social environment fulfills the need for attention and affection.

- Self-feeding is linked to a person's dignity, self-esteem, and relationships with others. Preserving feeding abilities is vital for the caregiving team. When disabilities limit self-feeding, maintain eye contact and conversation with the client during the feeding process.

- Monitor tablemates to ensure a positive interaction. To distinguish patterns, take note when clients become upset. If the client's pre-illness eating routine was solitary, then he or she may prefer to eat alone. Seat clients alone when they become agitated by others.

- Behavioral challenges such as agitation make mealtime more problematic. Observe for indications of behavioral changes that may interfere with eating. Modify the environment to discourage behavior changes. Catastrophic reactions can be evoked by subtle inconsistencies in the environment, such as a change in the place setting or a different seat.

- A successful mealtime includes a personalized approach with food preferences and a pleasant eating environment.

Audience Interaction for Slide 4-8

Ask the audience to describe how food and mealtimes impact their family, traditions, and memories.

Lecture Material for Slide 4-9

EATING AS AN ACTIVITY

As stated in previous modules, activities need to provide meaning and purpose. Making mealtime an activity boosts interest and enthusiasm. Remember that any purposeful activities enhance the client's quality of life.

- Involve the client with the entire process, not just the consumption of food. Meal planning, meal preparation, and setting the table are activities. The sense of accomplishment and success is achieved when including the client in the activity. For example, cooking and baking projects are purposeful activities with an enjoyable outcome.

- Address the client's food preferences whenever possible. The goal of this activity is to increase food and fluid intake while providing a successful activity. Incorporate a variety of foods into the client's diet. Plan meals that account for the individual's interest and traditions.

- Utilize all the principles to enhance a successful activity. Evaluate clients' functional level to determine what they can do, what they do, and how they do it. Since every client with AD is different, determining the level of functioning cannot be generalized.

- When performing mealtime tasks, highlight clients' abilities and strengths. Circumvent their weaknesses by developing alternate solutions. Praise all attempted appropriate activities. Use positive redirection without focusing on the failed segment of the task.

- Simple activities reinforce clients' self-esteem. Ensure the task is not too childlike or too advanced. Have them perform at their fullest potential.

- Avoid preconceived notions of the client's limitations. Observation needs to be objective. Limitations need to be foreseen, not presumed. Completing tasks for the client only causes a learned helplessness and degrades remaining skills. Learned helplessness occurs when the client has determined their efforts are futile. Institute changes when their ability to overcome barriers independently has diminished.

- Use behavioral and memory interventions to assist clients in achieving their highest level of independence. Montessori-based activities and space-retrieval practices can help clients learn and manage skills. See Module 2 for more information.

- The use of validation helps reduce the client's refusal to eat. Refusal to eat altogether may represent an effort on the part of the client to exert some control over their environment.

- Food trays are prepared with a predetermined diet and caloric count according to the client's needs. Clients should consume 75% or more of the meal. If more than 25% of the food remains, notify the supervisor.

- Ongoing evaluation ensures a pleasant and safe experience. Observe clients for their meal consumption, use of utensils, refusal of substitutions, loss of attentiveness, and difficulties with chewing and swallowing.

Lecture Material for Slide 4-10

● OBSERVATION AND REPORTING OF FEEDING PATTERNS

The caregiver must evaluate the client's ability in order for the individual to have a successful eating experience. Observing the client's ability to initiate a task, as well as the ability to respond to commands, helps determine the level of assistance required. Eating performance predicts and reflects outcomes in other activities. The goal of all interventions is to encourage the client to complete as much of the task as possible independently.

Feeding Assessment

The Feeding Abilities Assessment (FAA), developed by LeClerc and Wells, is useful in determining the highest level of functioning and minimizes learned dependence. The tool initially begins with a scenario that requires no assistance and rates the client's performance. Interventions are introduced only when the client is unsuccessful. Reevaluate the client's abilities routinely to maximize the chances of a successful activity.

The following summarizes the tool:

Observe the client's eating patterns for approximately two minutes to determine the client's ability to

- Initiate, sequence, and follow through with complex and simple motor actions.
- Use tools appropriately in complex and simple tasks.

The assessment takes place in parts:

1. This is the first part of the assessment. If the client is successful, no further interventions are needed. Place the food tray in front of the client and observe the client:
   - Pick up the utensil, remove the cover, and open all food wrappers.
   - Pick up the food with the utensils.
   - Bring the food to the mouth.
   - Continue the meal until full or finished.
   - Perform the actions in the correct sequence.
   - Choose and hold the appropriate utensil correctly.

2. If the client is unsuccessful, reduce the amount of decision making. Choose one food, with one utensil and no wrappers. Place a bowl of soup with a spoon in front of the client and observe the client:
   - Picking up the spoon.
   - Ladling the soup onto the spoon.
   - Bringing the spoon with the soup to the mouth.
   - Continuing until full or finished.

3. If the client continues to fail, incorporate minimal verbal prompting to assist the client with eating. The consequences of ideational

apraxia prevent the client from conceptualizing mealtime. Use prompts to remind the client of the purpose of the event.

- "It is time to eat your soup."
- "You are doing well."

4. Continue to add interventions until the client is successful. Use the task-breakdown technique to assist the client with eating. Prompt and demonstrate the activity to promote the completion of the task.

- "Pick up the spoon."
- "Put the spoon in the soup."
- "Bring the spoon to your mouth."

As the client's level of functioning deteriorates and feeding becomes increasingly challenging, observe the client with each additional intervention. Exhaust all self-feeding options prior to initiating hand-feeding.

Audience Interaction for Slide 4-10

Ask the audience for ways to promote independent eating with assistance. Include the following points in the discussion:

- Use gestures to assist clients with eating.
- Use verbal cues.
- Place the spoon in their hand.
- Guide their hand to ladle the soup.
- Use the hand-over-hand technique.

Insert agency's policy and procedure for documenting food and fluid intake here.

Lecture Material for Slide 4-11

EATING CHALLENGES

The cognitive deficit of clients with AD poses several eating challenges. Aspects of their social and physical environment can affect their dietary behaviors. Appropriate conditions improve their function and quality of life.

Special Dietary Needs

Clients may have special dietary needs resulting from previous medical conditions, such as hypoglycemia, diabetes, or food allergies, which present challenges. The caregiver must monitor clients' dietary habits, since their judgment is impaired.

- Small frequent meals help manage clients with hypoglycemia and diabetes. The caregiver may limit the types of snacks offered to better control their diet. Diabetic clients respond well when they eat the same amount of food at the same time each day. Skipping meals, eating at different times, or eating concentrated sweets makes keeping blood sugar under control difficult.

- Small frequent meals decreases a variety of common gastric symptoms.
- Staff should be notified of all clients with food allergies. Medical identification tags need to be worn by clients. Communicating the allergy to visitors is appropriate when food is brought in for special events. Post a generic sign stressing that visitors notify staff of all incoming food.
- Unmonitored snacking can affect clients on special diets (diabetic diet, low cholesterol, low sodium) and may lead to potentially harmful conditions.

Hoarding Food

Hoarding, a common behavior among AD clients, represents cognitive impairment. The hoarding of food can create feelings of security. Discarding items requires decision-making skills, which they no longer possess. Clients may not be able to determine, for example, that the banana peel is not edible. Hoarding food can cause safety and health hazards. Clients may be unaware they are hoarding the items.

- Observe clients' snacking habits to assure they are within the limits of their diet. Compulsive snacking of non-nutritious foods reduces healthy eating at regular mealtimes.
- Foods are habitually hidden in the same spot. Routinely check clients' rooms for saved food. To diminish anxiety, leave a few of the items, when appropriate, as long as the food will not spoil or attract bugs. Reassure the individual that food is available.
- When saving foods, store them in a closed container. Frequently remind clients of the location of their "stash" to reduce the taking of additional items. Monitor the snacks to assure that clients are not trading stale or perished snacks with others.

Over and Undereating

Memory loss, poor judgment, and no longer understanding the feeling of being full are possible causes for clients with dementia to under or overeat. Previous eating habits may also come into play. The role food played in the individual's pre-illness life remains through the early stages of the disease.

- The client's weight should be routinely monitored. Notify the supervisor of any changes in weight. As stated previously, medical conditions may impact the client's food intake and should be investigated prior to changes in the plan.
- Agitation, restlessness, pacing, or other calorie-burning activities can cause weight loss. Additional nutritious snacks may be necessary. Clients may need foods, which can be eaten "on the run" when behaviors such as wandering are part of their routine.
- If depression is the cause of the client's anorexia, introducing antidepressants may help diminish the weight loss.

- Liquid calorie supplements are available to help underweight clients or those who do not enjoy eating food. Including homemade foods from the family may encourage clients to eat. Protein drinks, yogurt, and milk shakes can be used as snacks to increase calories.
- Overeating may be due to boredom. Increase the client's level of socialization and activities to break the pattern.
- When necessary, lock cupboards or pantries to limit food accessibility.
- When weight gain is an issue, offer low-calorie snacks and beverages.

Eating Inedible Objects

- Dementia clients have difficulty distinguishing the difference between edible and inedible foods. Occasionally a client may mistake dirt in a flowerpot, decorative soap, pet food, or cleaning implements for food.
- The desire to consume these products is the result of altered decision-making skills. The items must be kept out of sight if they become problematic.
- Remove condiments from the client's eating area. The client may or may not be able to determine their use and consume them as if they were a food choice. Most clients with cognitive impairment get increasingly confused when faced with multiple condiments on the table.

Accusations of Stealing Food

- Suspiciousness is a commonly observed behavior in the latter stages of the disease. The behavior is attributed to a faltering memory and/or an inability to recognize friends and family. Fear is usually the underlying reason for all accusations.
- The caregiver's goal is to restore order when suspicious behaviors occur. Determine if the accusations are true or false. The caregiver needs to protect clients when their fears are factual. They may complain that someone is stealing their food, when in fact another resident does eat the cookies the family leaves.
- Another interpretation of the accusations is that the client remains hungry and is unable to verbalize the hunger.

● EATING SAFETY

Lecture Material for Slide 4-12

Mealtime presents many potential hazards and requires careful evaluation of the plan of care. The client's impaired judgment can lead to potential injuries, behavioral challenges, and medical conditions related to poor nutrition.

Observation

Ongoing assessment is an essential part of the care planning process.

- Clients with dementia can perform some tasks on some days and not on others. Observing the client's ability during mealtime and adjusting the interventions as needed promote the optimal level of nutritional intake.

- Assist the client with eating to promote independence as well as to prevent aspiration or choking.
- The client's overall mood may affect his or her safety when eating. Anxious clients may choke on their food or may not thoroughly chew all their food before taking another bite.
- The client may have suffered loss of coordination and is unable to hold utensils. The supervisor or therapist can demonstrate the use of adaptive eating devices.
- Ask the supervisor if the client has difficulty swallowing (dysphagia). Normal swallowing takes less than two seconds to move the food from the mouth to the esophagus. Assess swallowing before meals. Avoid foods prone to producing choking such as popcorn, nuts, and sticky foods.

Eating Position

Safe eating requires the body to be positioned in a proper alignment for swallowing and ingesting food:

- The client sits upright with the body and the head bent slightly forward.
- The knees are bent and the feet are flat on the floor.
- The head is tilted forward to assist with swallowing.
- Properly place the food on the plate for easy visualization.
- Have the client remain in the forward position (head upright and leaning forward) until all the food in the mouth has been cleared.

Have the client remain seated for 10 to 15 minutes following the meal. Movement immediately following eating may precipitate vomiting or indigestion.

Medical Conditions Caused by Feeding Problems

Medical conditions can result when a client has problems with eating. Most often, the problems stem from the individual's inability to swallow food and fluids.

Aspiration

Aspiration is the inhaling of food, saliva, or stomach contents into the lungs, usually resulting in pneumonia. Aspiration pneumonia can be treated with antibiotics, but frequently results in a reoccurrence of pneumonia requiring hospitalization.

Dehydration

Dehydration is the excessive loss of water from the body tissues. Dehydration is accompanied by a disturbance in the balance of essential electrolytes. When the client is unable to swallow liquids, the body becomes dehydrated.

Malnutrition

Malnutrition is any disorder affecting the necessary nutrients for body cells. It may result from an unbalanced, insufficient, radical diet or from impairments in the absorption of food. When food intake is reduced due to difficulties with swallowing, the client becomes malnourished without intervention.

Dysphagia

Dysphagia is difficulty in swallowing commonly associated with obstructive or motor disorders of the esophagus. Comorbid conditions, such as Parkinson's disease, multiple sclerosis, and stroke, may contribute to the condition.

Causes of Swallowing Problems

- Difficulty closing the lips and mouth.
- Difficulty moving the tongue to control food to chew or to push food to the back of the mouth.
- Weakness in the facial muscles, causing a collection of food in the cheeks (food pocketing).
- Loss of sensation in the mouth and an inability to feel the location of the food in the mouth.
- The inability to trigger the pharynx muscles to assist with swallowing.
- Difficulty coordinating the muscles to close the larynx.
- Damage to the muscles in the pharynx, causing food to be left in the throat.
- The inability of esophageal muscles to move food down the esophagus.

SIGNS OF DYSPHAGIA

Some clients may not exhibit outward signs of dysphagia. A swallowing test, performed prior to eating a normal diet, determines whether a swallowing problem exists. Notify the supervisor of any signs of dysphagia.

Commonly Observed Signs of Dysphagia

- Coughing while eating or drinking.
- A wet sounding voice during or after eating.
- Increased congestion in the chest after eating or drinking.
- Slow eating.
- Multiple swallows on one mouthful of food.
- Effort or difficulty while chewing or swallowing.
- Fatigue or shortness of breath (SOB) while eating.
- Fever or a rise in body temperature 30 minutes to one hour after eating.

- Weight loss.
- Frequent pneumonia.

Dysphagia Diets

Dysphagia diets are used when clients have difficulty swallowing. The diets are based on food consistency. The dysphagia diet includes blenderized and semiliquid foods requiring no chewing and are easy to swallow. Food consistency is modified according to the individual's swallowing ability.

- If they can manage, give clients food that can be chewed. One piece of food is easier to eat than many small pieces. Avoid foods that easily break apart (eg, rice or chopped meats).
- The client's gag reflex should be evaluated before introducing certain foods.
- Thin liquids, such as milk, juice, coffee, tea, soda, and broth, are excluded unless specifically recommended or ordered as thickened liquids. Thickened liquids are ordered with different thickness levels, such as honey thickened, nectar thickened, or pudding thickened.
- Water, milk, juice, broth, plain gravies, and sauces may be used to thin foods to the desired consistency or to moisten them for easier swallowing.
- Blenderized meat, cooked cereal, pureed vegetables and fruits, mashed potatoes, and yogurt may be used as thickening agents. Commercial thickening agents are available, or already thickened water, milk, and fruit juices can be purchased at the thickness required.
- Thickening by adding butter, margarine, sugar, or honey to food can also furnish additional calories, assuming no dietary restrictions exist.
- Cook food with eggs as an ingredient to provide thickness and additional nutrients.

Lecture Material for Slides 4-15 and 4-16

Slide 4-15

ORAL FEEDINGS VERSUS TUBE FEEDINGS

During the latter stages of Alzheimer's disease, clients become dependent in all areas of activities of daily living, including eating. Families are then faced with the burden of choosing to continue oral feedings or to initiate tube feedings.

- Swallowing and eating problems are the hallmarks of end-stage AD. Problems stem from the inability to swallow (similar to stroke victims), the inability to self-feed, or the lack of interest in food.
- When the client is no longer ingesting food, a controversial decision needs to be made on whether or not to insert a feeding tube. Decisions regarding end-of-life care should be discussed early on in the disease to lessen the burden for families.

Oral Feedings

- Continuing oral feedings as long as it is enjoyable and comfortable for clients is recommended by the medical community. The staff should increase opportunities for clients to ingest food and fluids.
- Once clients are no longer able to self-feed, they can be hand-fed. Hand-feeding is a nurturing intervention, providing social interaction. Use the hand-over-hand technique. Place the person's hand around an object, such as a glass, and then the caregiver's hand goes over the client's hand and guides the glass to the client's mouth.
- Nutritional care should focus on comfort and palliative measures when clients are in the final stages of the disease.
- The literature suggests that individuals at the end of life no longer experience hunger or thirst. Most of their symptoms may be alleviated with proper mouth care and ice chips.

Audience Interaction for Slide 4-15

Ask the audience for ways to increase a client's food and fluid intake. Include the following in the discussion: nutritional supplements, adjusting textures and portion size, hand-feeding, special diets, social gatherings, and "happy hours."

Slide 4-16

Tube Feedings

A tube feeding is the administration of nutritionally balanced liquefied foods through a tube inserted into the stomach. When a client is unable to ingest, chew, or swallow, but is still able to digest and absorb food, tube feedings may be initiated.

- The feeding tube can be placed in the esophagus, stomach, or upper small intestine.
- Over 50% of nursing home clients with dementia are tube fed.
- All risks and benefits should be explained to families prior to the insertion of a feeding tube.
- Some studies have shown no difference in survival between clients who are tube fed and those receiving only palliative care. Also, no significant improvement in weight gain was found after tube feedings were initiated in dementia clients.

Potential Risks Associated with Tube Feedings

Tube feedings do not reduce the risk of pressure ulcers or aspiration. They may pose additional risks for clients, such as:

- Infection.
- Dislodgment of tube.
- Gastrointestinal disturbances (diarrhea, nausea, and vomiting).
- Hospitalization.
- Aspiration.
- Increased use of restraints (used to prevent clients from pulling out tubes).

In the end, the primary goal is to treat clients with respect and dignity. No matter the feeding method, all clients' nutritional status must be routinely evaluated. Ongoing observation and reporting are essential. Caregivers must remain objective regardless of their personal beliefs or wishes regarding oral and tube feedings.

Lecture Material for Slides 4-17 and 4-18

Slide 4-17

ASSISTING WITH FEEDINGS

Individuals with dementia can remain independent with feeding and enjoy its social aspects by incorporating interventions into the plan of care. Caregivers need to make mealtime a person-centered, not a staff-centered, activity.

Ways to Assist Clients' with Feeding

- Observation and reporting.
- Verbal cues and prompting.
- Gestures.
- Partial physical assistance.
- Total physical assistance.

Slide 4-18

Things to Know

- Speak slowly and clearly when giving instructions to clients. Be consistent and repeat instructions with the same words each time.
- Use distractions when clients begin to exhibit challenging behaviors.
- Use memory aids to remind clients to eat and drink.
- To open a person's mouth, ask the person to say "ah" or yawn. Applying slight pressure to the chin aids in opening a client's mouth.
- Use plates with no patterns to compensate for visual perception difficulties.
- Use a place mat with dual-sided rubber to prevent plate movement.
- Use bowls whenever possible, as opposed to plates, for a more successful eating experience. Altered coordination skills may hinder a client's ability to spear the foods with utensils.
- Adaptive eating devices are available to help the client with eating.
- Use rubber-coated utensils if the client is biting too hard.
- Encourage the use of spoons; they are easier than forks to manipulate.
- The use of plastic utensils is not recommended. The utensils are lightweight and may break in the client's mouth.
- Use bendable straws or lidded cups for liquids. Replace soup bowls with mugs for ease. Cups with handles are easier to use.

- Reposition foods during meals as often as needed to increase intake.
- Encourage fluids by offering sherbet, Popsicles®, gelatin, or slushies.
- Use multisensory cueing to enhance the cognitive memories of mealtimes.
- Encourage clients to wear their corrective glasses, hearing aids, and dentures.
- Encourage conversation.
- Sit with the client when prompting and assisting with eating.
- Maintain eye contact with the client when assisting with feedings.
- Offer prayer or a moment of silence before meals, as appropriate.
- Offer reassurance and verbal praise for positive behaviors.
- Assess the client's need for pain management.
- Encourage proper oral care.
- Most importantly, remain patient. The client's food and fluid preferences may change frequently, and mealtime may last for an hour or more.

SUMMING UP

As Alzheimer's disease progresses and consumes more of the individual's intellect, nutrition and eating challenges develop. The once simple task of eating becomes impeded by the inability to go through the intricate sequences needed to: locate the dining room, understand the sensation of hunger and thirst, utilize the tableware, visually see food on the plate, have motor coordination, chew, and swallow. Weight fluctuations can result from memory loss, confusion, communication skills, and changes in caloric demand. Previous eating habits also impact eating problems.

The plan of care should support the client's physical health, physical environment, and social environment. The plan should be person-centered, taking a personalized approach with food preferences and customs. Interventions can be implemented to prolong the ability to eat and to provide successful, meaningful activities for the client and family. Eating behaviors can be improved by utilizing behavioral strategies. The nutritional goal for the client with dementia is to provide well-balanced meals and snacks. Observation and reporting the client's feeding patterns help to bolster strengths and assist with weakness while encouraging independence. Eating challenges, such as special diets, hoarding food, or eating inedible objects, can be addressed within the plan of care.

When clients approach the latter stages of the disease, they no longer feed. Eating and swallowing are the last skills to be lost in the course of the illness. Clients become unable to swallow and run the risk of aspiration and other medical conditions. Families are faced with the decision whether to continue oral feeding or initiate tube feeding.

Module 4 **EATING CHALLENGES WITH DEMENTIA** 153

Instructor's Version with Answers for Handout 4-2

● REAL-LIFE SCENARIO

A Day in the Life of Pat

Pat has always been a hearty eater, even after relocating to the Sunny Brook Nursing Home. Recently, Pat has been eating less. According to the meal intake documentation form completed by the staff at each meal, Pat is consuming less than 30% of the meal.

1. What should the caregiver be observing during mealtime?

    The caregiver should be observing Pat's:
    - *Reaction when the meal tray is placed in front of Pat.*
    - *Ability to access the food.*
    - *Ability to properly use the utensils.*
    - *Ability to visualize the food on the plate.*
    - *Ability to chew and swallow.*
    - *Attention span while eating.*
    - *Interaction with others at the table.*
    - *Food preferences.*

    The caregiver should also be aware of any changes in the environment, behavioral changes, changes in medication, or medical conditions.

2. What type of eating challenges do caregivers face with dementia clients?

    Caregivers are faced with the following eating challenges when caring for clients with dementia:
    - *Keeping clients on special diets.*
    - *Hoarding food.*
    - *Over and undereating.*
    - *Eating inedible objects.*
    - *Accusations of stealing food.*

3. List five ways the caregiver can maintain a supportive physical environment for eating.

    The caregiver can maintain a supportive physical environment for eating by:
    - *Maintaining routines.*
    - *Using visual cues.*
    - *Limiting noise.*
    - *Maintaining a pleasant eating atmosphere.*
    - *Adjusting seating as necessary.*
    - *Using contrasting colors.*
    - *Using modified and assistive devices.*
    - *Reviewing food selections.*
    - *Using verbal cues and prompts.*

GROUP ACTIVITY

● PURPOSE OF THE ACTIVITY

The purpose of this activity is to reinforce interventions to support dementia clients during mealtime. The following activities can be completed as a class, in small groups, or individually.

Option 1

Make a list of interventions that support a client with dementia during mealtime. Utilize all elements to promote a successful activity for the client. The following should be addressed in the answer: table setting, seating, atmosphere, food choices, tablemates, meal planning, choking, caregiver support, and oral care.

Option 2

Role-play common "difficult moments" exhibited during mealtime. Possible scenarios may include refusing to go to the dining hall, being unable to sit down in the chair, or attempting to eat nonfood items. Discuss solutions and alternative ways to handle the scenario. Reverse roles with other "difficult moments."

Name _____ Date _____

Program/Course _____ Instructor's Name _____

Eating Challenges with Dementia Pre- and Post-Test

1. What are the hallmarks of end-stage Alzheimer's disease?
   a. Tangles and plaques.
   b. Inability to speak and communicate.
   c. Swallowing and eating problems.
   d. Loss of bowel and bladder function.

2. Ideational apraxia is defined as:
   a. The loss of the ability to conceptualize, plan, prepare, and implement the intricate sequences of complex motor tasks involving objects, regardless of muscle sensation and coordination.
   b. Difficulty in swallowing associated with obstructive or motor disorders of the esophagus.
   c. A condition characterized by the refusal to eat or swallow because doing so causes pain.
   d. An abnormal neurologic condition in which language function is defective.

3. Dysphagia is defined as:
   a. The impaired ability to perform purposeful acts or to manipulate objects.
   b. Difficulty in swallowing associated with obstructive or motor disorders of the esophagus.
   c. A condition characterized by the refusal to eat or swallow because doing so causes pain.
   d. An abnormal neurologic condition in which language function is defective.

4. What should a caregiver observe the client for during mealtime?
   a. Meal consumption, the use of utensils, and the refusal of food substitutions.
   b. The loss of attentiveness and difficulties with chewing and swallowing.
   c. Both A and B.
   d. Neither A or B.

(continued)

Handout **4-1**

Eating Challenges with Dementia Pre- and Post-Test (Continued)

5. What are four ways to increase a client's food and fluid intake?
   a. Singing, dancing, running, and playing.
   b. Incorporating spices, thickening agents, ice cream, and rice into the diet.
   c. Smaller portion sizes, frequent meals, force feeding, and high-fat foods.
   d. Nutritional supplements, social gatherings, and adjusting food textures and portion size.

A Day in the Life of Pat: A Real-Life Scenario

Pat has always been a hearty eater, even after relocating to the Sunny Brook Nursing Home. Recently, Pat has been eating less. According to the meal intake documentation form completed by the staff at each meal, Pat is consuming less than 30% of the meal.

1. What should the caregiver be observing during mealtime?

2. What type of eating challenges do caregivers face with dementia clients?

3. List five ways the caregiver can maintain a supportive physical environment for eating.

Handout **4-2**

MODULE 4 EATING CHALLENGES WITH DEMENTIA

Cognitive Impairments Leading to Eating Challenges

- **Memory loss and confusion**
- **Inability to recognize sensations**
- **Impaired thought process**
- **Loss of senses**

Cognitive Impairments Leading to Eating Challenges (cont.)

- **Neuromuscular dyscoordination**
- **Visual changes**
- **Changes in communication skills**
- **Apraxia**

Eating Challenges Due to Ideational Apraxia

- **Not eating the food in front of them**
- **Mixing foods**
- **Using the incorrect utensil**

Eating Challenges Due to Ideational Apraxia (*cont.*)

- **Eating foods still in the wrapper**
- **Eating inedible objects**
- **Incorrect eating sequence**

Maintaining a Supportive Physical Environment

- **Maintain routines**
- **Use visual cues**
- **Limit noise**
- **Maintain a pleasant eating atmosphere**
- **Adjust seating as necessary**

Maintaining a Supportive Physical Environment (*cont.*)

- **Use contrasting colors**
- **Use modified and assistive devices**
- **Review food selections**
- **Use verbal cues and prompts**

Maintaining a Supportive Social Environment

- **Promote communication skills**
- **Maintain calmness**
- **Encourage socialization**
- **Preserve feeding abilities**
- **Review seating arrangements**
- **Personalize mealtime**

Eating as an Activity

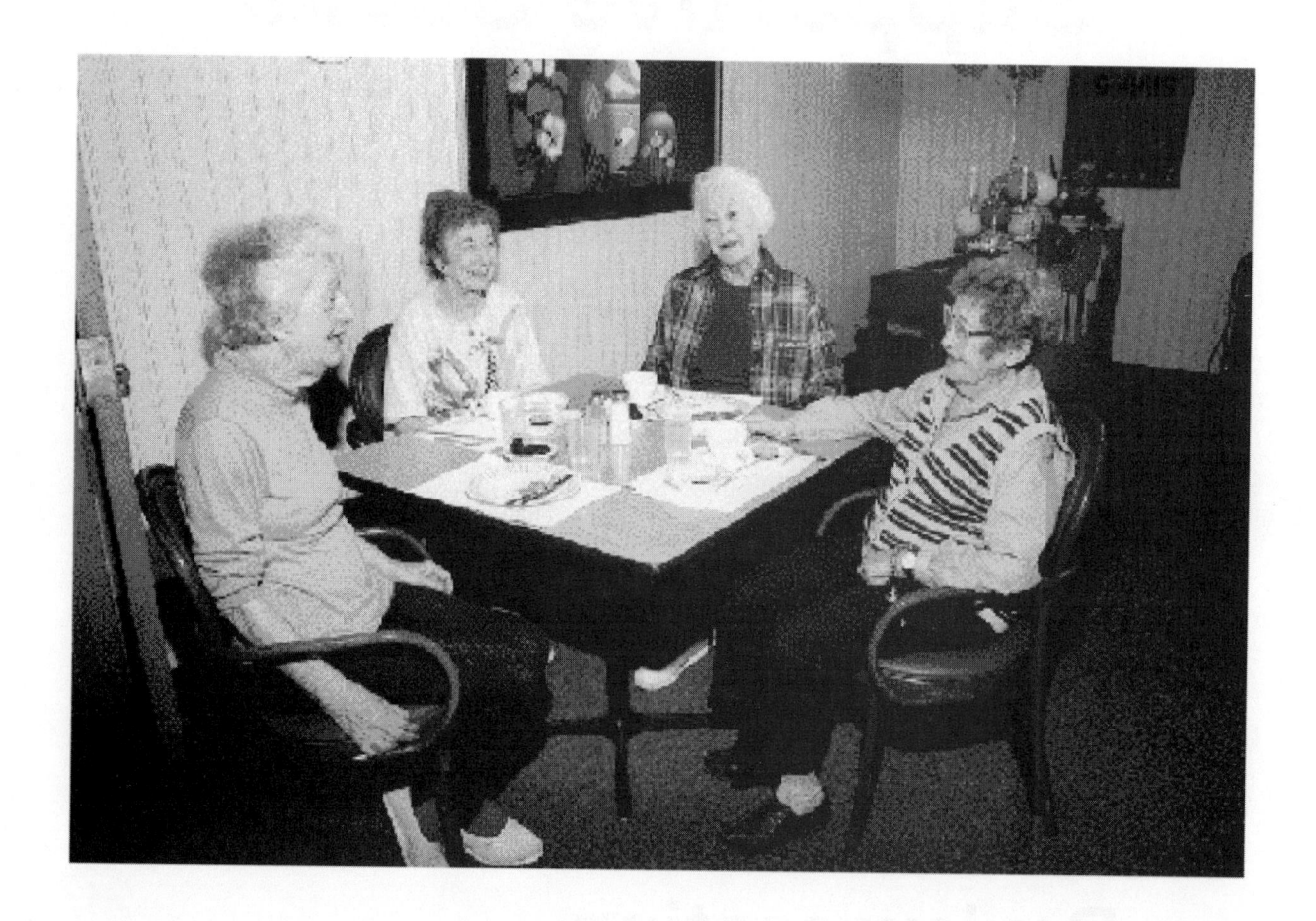

Observation and Reporting Feeding Patterns

- **Initiate eating**
- **Eating sequence**
- **Follow through of eating actions**
- **The correct use of utensils**

Eating Challenges

- **Special diets**
- **Hoarding food**
- **Over- and under-eating**
- **Eating inedible objects**
- **Accusations of stealing food**

! CAUTION Eating Safety

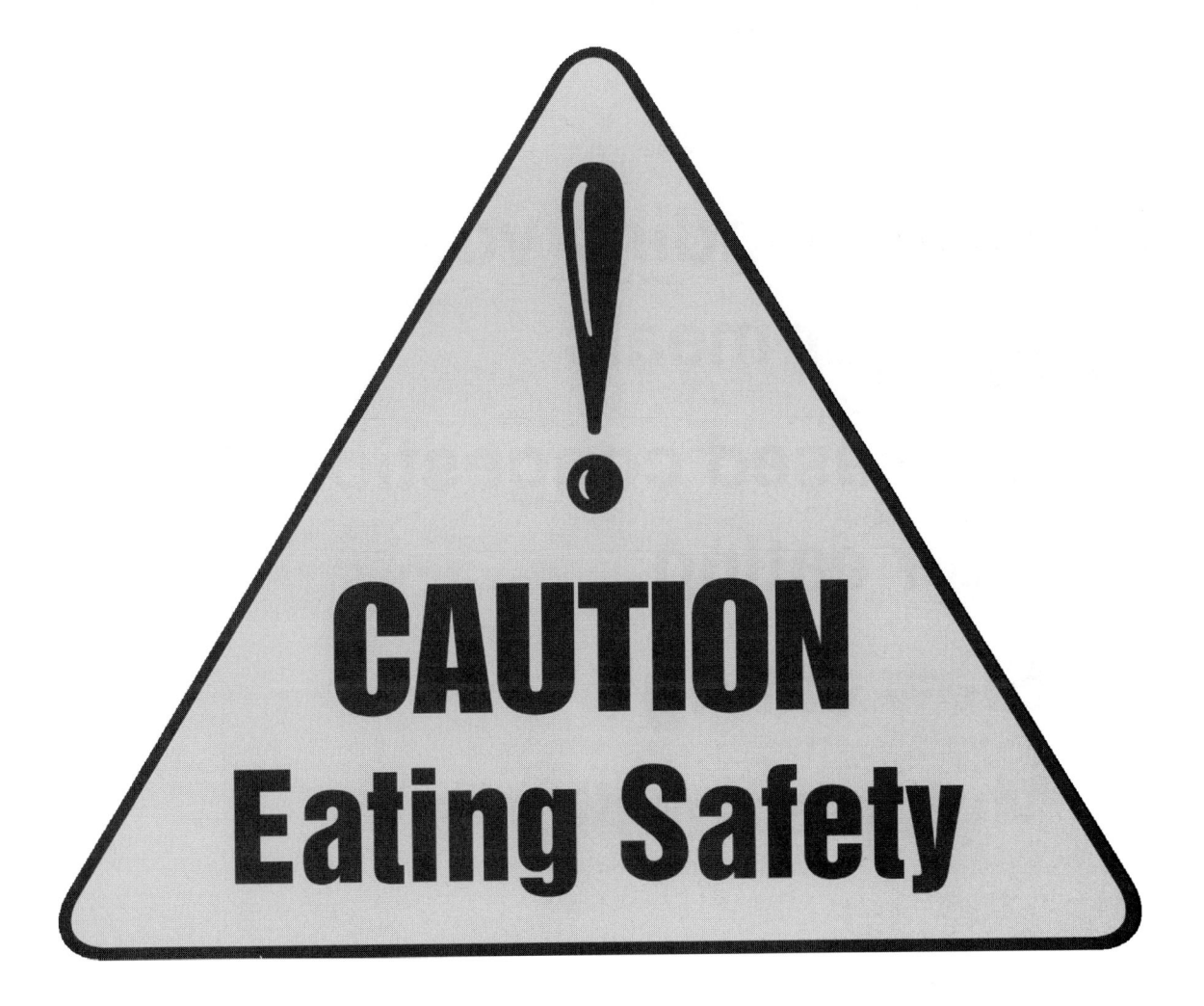

Signs of Dysphagia

- **Coughing during eating or drinking**
- **Wet sounding voice during or after meals**
- **Increased congestion after eating**
- **Slow eating**
- **Multiple swallows**

Signs of Dysphagia (cont.)

- **Difficulty chewing or swallowing**
- **Fatigue or SOB when eating**
- **Fever**
- **Weight loss**
- **Pneumonia**

Oral feedings vs. Tube feedings

Potential Risks of Tube Feedings

- **Infection**
- **Dislodgment of tube**
- **GI disturbances**
- **Hospitalization**
- **Aspiration**
- **Increased use of restraints**

Ways to Assist with Feeding

- **Observation and reporting**
- **Verbal cues and prompting**
- **Partial physical assistance**
- **Total physical assistance**

Module 4 **EATING CHALLENGES WITH DEMENTIA** 175

Things to Know

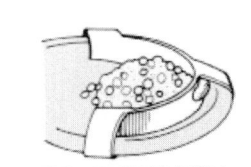

A. PLATE GUARD SNAPS OVER A DINNER PLATE TO KEEP THE FOOD ON THE PLATE.

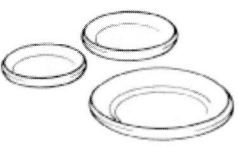

B. PLATES WITH INNER LIP TO KEEP FOOD ON PLATE.

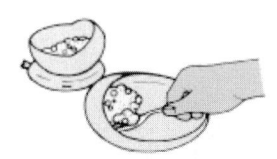

C. PLATE WITH HIGH CURVED EDGE TO HELP PUSH FOOD ON FORK OR SPOON.

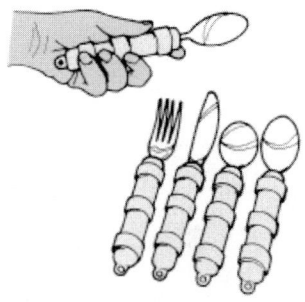

D. CUTLERY WITH BUILT-UP HANDLES FOR EASIER GRIPPING; MOVABLE GRIP RINGS ADJUST FOR COMFORT.

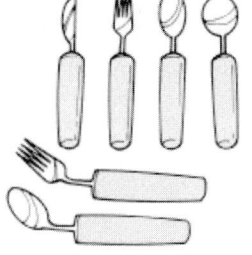

E. ANGLED CUTLERY FOR PEOPLE WITH LIMITED ARM AND WRIST MOVEMENT.

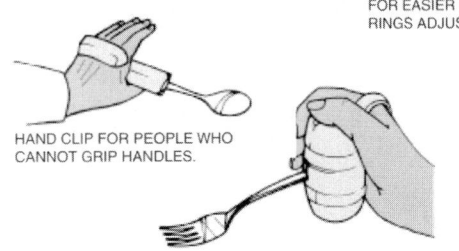

HAND CLIP FOR PEOPLE WHO CANNOT GRIP HANDLES.

F. GRIPPER FOR PEOPLE WHO CANNOT GRIP STANDARD OR BUILT-UP HANDLES.

Transparency Master **4-18**

Copyright © 2007 by Delmar Learning, a division of Thomson Learning, Inc.

Module 5
Recreation and Activities

Goal

To better understand how to manage activities for the cognitively impaired client.

Objectives

After the completion of the presentation, students will be able to:

- List seven ways purposeful activities enhance a client's quality of life.
- Describe what cognitive functions are needed to complete complex tasks.
- Explain the memory process.
- List Zgola's (1987) seven Ws of a function evaluation.
- Describe reasons for wandering.
- List five ways to prevent falls.
- Describe the features of a successful activity.

Lecture Material for Slide 5-1

GENERAL INFORMATION/OVERVIEW

Alzheimer's disease is a complex disorder that is particularly challenging to treat and manage. While the disease progresses, it is marked by unrelenting cognitive and functional decline, and it can impose a significant burden on families and caregivers. The simplest tasks become obstacles to the dementia client. Theories suggest losing the ability to complete tasks and maintain roles erodes the person's identity. The repeated unsuccessfulness of activities creates more boundaries and causes withdrawal from society. The complex nature of each individual is affected by the physical condition of Alzheimer's disease.

- The progression of Alzheimer's symptoms can take from two to 20 years, with an average life span of eight to 10 years from diagnosis. During this time everyday tasks like bathing and dressing become more and more difficult.

- All human beings have a fundamental psychological need to be active. However, the nerve pathways in the brain, which are associated with motivation, may be damaged in a person with dementia. Any recreational plans need to incorporate interventions that focus on ways to initiate tasks.

- Researchers suggest that participation in leisure activities has been associated with a lower risk of dementia.

- Studies conclude that incorporating programs involving exercise and behavior techniques among clients with AD resulted in an increased physical activity level, less depression, and improved physical health and function.

- Having a greater intellectual resource may buffer the underlying damage associated with the early stages of dementia, hence delaying the onset of symptoms.

- Continuous involvement in purposeful mental activities may promote changes in the brain that circumvent the pathology underlying the symptoms of dementia. Mental activity may not only strengthen existing synaptic connections and generate new ones, but also stimulate neurogenesis, especially in the hippocampus. (Coyle, 2003)

- In America, more than 34,000 Alzheimer's clients are reported to wander out of their homes or care facilities each year. (Warner, 2002)

- Nationally, 70% of negligence claims to insurance companies regarding clients who have wandered away from residential facilities are filed because wandering resulted in death. (Flaherty, 2002)

Lecture Material for Slides 5-2 and 5-3

Slide 5-2

ACTIVITIES

Activities define a person, allowing individuals to exert control over their environment. The participation in activities provides relationships with others and fulfills most psychosocial needs. Everyone has a basic human need for activity and rest. Activity also provides the physical stresses needed for normal cell growth and development.

When a disease process develops a person's level of participation in and the types of activities change. The loss of cognitive function, as seen in AD clients, is not always obvious to others. With cognitive impairments, clients' needs for assistance are often ignored or possibly ridiculed. They may become reluctant or even hostile when asked to complete a task for fear of revealing their deficits. Reactions to the obviously sick or ill are very different from the typical reaction to persons with AD. The limitations of evidently ill clients are noticeable to everyone, and plans to address their needs are easily established. This is not so true for clients with dementia.

Activities can be grouped into three categories: productive, leisure, and self-care. Each has an impact on the person's sense of self. Always remember that any purposeful activities improve the quality of life for the client.

- Make sure the activity is person-centered. As mentioned previously, learning about the client through interviews with the family (or the client's medical record) enhances any activity program by taking into account the individual's interest and traditions.

The Benefits of Purposeful Activities

Purposeful activities:

- Enhance feelings of self-worth.
- Create enjoyment.
- Promote general health.
- Preserve memory.
- Maintain communication skills.
- Improve personal relationships.
- Promote family interactions.
- Increase muscle strength and flexibility.
- Reduce nervous tension.
- Decrease pacing and restlessness.
- Reduce wandering.
- Increase nighttime sleep.

Slide 5-3

Utilize this time to review the functions of the brain and the necessary cognitive abilities needed to complete tasks. (Review Handout 1-2 for more information.)

Lecture Material for Slide 5-4

● COGNITIVE ABILITIES NEEDED TO COMPLETE TASKS

Changes in the cerebral cortex of the brain cause the AD client to fail at the simplest of tasks. Each chore, duty, or assignment completed requires multiple functions from the brain.

The following cognitive functions are required for all individuals to complete an activity successfully.

Language

- Forming words into sentences in order to communicate is an unconscious process for most people.
- The person with dementia, along with other brain injured clients, suffers from language difficulties.

See Module 2 for detailed lecture material.

Memory

- Memory is the ability to store and recall previous experiences. Learning and memory are therefore inseparable processes.
- Learning involves comparing new experiences with remembered experiences and gaining a new understanding.
- Memories are stored in one area of the brain. Long-term memory may be archived by more than a single mechanism.
- Memory itself is very complex and involves a combination of brain pathways.

Types of Memory

- Primary, or immediate, memory is the recall of small bits of information lasting for a few seconds to a few minutes. This type of memory has a very limited capacity in how long the items are stored. An example is remembering a phone number long enough to dial the phone number.
- Recent memory measures the ability of the client to remember events occurring the same day.
- Remote memory involves remembering things that happened in the distant past (months to years). Remote memory is retained during much of AD.
- Semantic memory refers to the accumulation of facts and experiences over a lifetime.
- Sensory memory is the retention of actual sensory images in the sensory area of the brain. Individuals favor different senses and remember material experienced through that particular sense. For example, the ability to recall the landscape after looking out the window is utilizing the sensory memory of sight, or the sound of the ocean may bring back memories of the beach from childhood.

Creating a Memory

- Encoding is the first step in creating memories. Sensations travel to specific parts of the brain and integrate the perceptions into single experiences.

- Once a memory is created, it must be stored. All information does not need to be stored permanently. The brain sorts the information and determines if the memories should be kept short-term or long-term. The creation of a memory begins with the person's perception.
- After using or frequently thinking about an item, event, phrase, or person, the information becomes part of short-term memory and later part of long-term memory.
- Retaining is the process of converting short-term memory into long-term memory.
- As a person learns and remembers, the connections between new cells are reinforced.

Problems with Creating a Memory

Problems can take place at any point in the process of formulating a memory.
- The person with dementia may not be able to respond to a memory because the material did not register (lack of attention).
- The brain may no longer have the ability to perceive the information as important and does not store the data.
- The dying brain cells are unable to develop pathways to store details. Problems with storing short-term memories are common with all forms of dementia.
- The retrieval of information can be very frustrating to clients because they are acutely aware of their inability to remember.
- The storage of information may only be for a limited period of time.

Abstract Thought

- Interpreting abstract ideas or concepts reflects the capacity for abstract thinking. The person with AD may take phrases literally, causing misunderstandings.
- A higher level of intellectual functioning is required for an individual to explain proverbs such as "a stitch in time saves nine" or commands like "make the bed."

Organization

- Organizing thoughts to complete tasks requires a multitude of actions from the brain. With dementia, the brain no longer can process numerous thoughts simultaneously.
- Skilled movements require translating ideas into motor actions, organizing actions and events in a logical sequence, and then bringing everything together to complete the task.
- For example, the series of details needed to make a bed includes not only the organization of the bed linens, but also the coordination of movements of the individual.

Perception

- Perception is the process through which sensory information is recognized and interpreted. The input of information and the cognitive interpretation of data are both required for an individual to perceive an idea.
- The most common perceptual problem associated with AD is visuospatial difficulties: the inability to perceive direction, distance, and the spatial relationship of objects to one's body and to each other.
- Deficits in perception may cause the client to become lost.
- The client may be unable to distinguish between markings on a flat surface or to judge distance.

Attention

- Attention requires the concentration of mental powers on an object, with close or careful observation or listening.
- The initiation and continuation of a task require attention.
- The ability to concentrate is hindered by the effects of Alzheimer's disease, as witnessed in the client's lack of focus.
- Many problematic behaviors are caused by the client's loss of attention. Clients no longer have the initiative to start activities. Their attention span, or the length of time during which they can concentrate on a subject or idea, is markedly diminished. Clients have difficulty staying with the task once it has been started.
- The client may also get "stuck" in a pattern of behavior (perseveration): for example, rewashing the same glass over and over until something or someone brings the activity to a stop.

Judgment

- Judgment is a term encompassing all the cognition involving the process of evaluation, assessment, and decision making.
- Judgment requires a comparison and evaluation of facts and ideas to understand the relationships and to form appropriate conclusions.
- Individuals with impaired judgment may exhibit behaviors lacking regard for social etiquette.

MAKING AN ACTIVITY SUCCESSFUL

Lecture Material for Slide 5-5

The purpose of a successful activity is to increase an individual's confidence. Remember that clients are surrounded by failure. Simple activities reinforce their self-esteem, in addition to relieving boredom and providing purpose. Make sure the activity is not too childlike or to advanced for them.

Promote Strengths

Develop activities geared to clients' strengths and weakness. They should perform at their fullest potential.

- Clients with dementia can perform some tasks on some days and not on others. Even the time of day can produce fluctuations in functioning. This can be disconcerting to caregivers and frustrating to clients.
- Knowing clients' strengths can lessen disappointment by encouraging them to perform a previously successful task. Since they are not able to retain the memory of the failed activity, they can enjoy the current task.

Maintain Goals

Incorporate all aspects of the client's plan of care into a successful activity. Interventions that support each of the three care plan goals (maintaining physical health, physical environment, and social environment) can make for purposeful activities.

- Goals are based on maximizing clients' current abilities and preventing deterioration.
- Activities should reflect their likes and dislikes. The chosen activities reinforce the goals of the plan of care.
- Use a person-centered approach when formulating activities and duties.

Observation and Reporting

As stressed in previous modules, the importance of ongoing evaluation is an essential part of the care planning process. On the first encounter with the client, take a virtual snapshot photo of him or her. Determine if it matches the information given in the report about the client. Use the information as the baseline and compare the client's progress. Report any changes in the client's condition to the supervisor immediately.

- Be objective when observing the client. Many stereotypes about AD can create preconceived notions of the client's limitations. A false assumption that a client is unable to accomplish tasks causes a learned helplessness on the client's part and degrades any skills the client may retain.
- Limitations should be foreseen but not presumed. Reassess the client's inability to overcome limitations independently and act accordingly.

● FUNCTIONAL EVALUATION

The evaluation, developed by Jitka Zgola, is used to determine what the client can do, what the client does, and how the client does it. Since every client with AD is different, determining the level of functioning cannot be generalized. Many times a client performs at a higher level than the neuropsychological testing predicts. The framework poses the seven Ws, questions to help assess the client's level of functioning.

Zgola's Seven Ws of a Functional Evaluation

- What can the client do?
- What does the client do?
- How does he or she do it?
- Which parts of the task is the client unable to do?
- Why is he or she unable to do them?
- Where does he or she perform best?
- When does he or she perform best?

Slide 5-7

Components of a Functional Evaluation

All aspects of the individual are reviewed through each component of the evaluation to help establish the best plan possible. A functional evaluation outlines the client's level of independent living, mobility, senses and functions, self-care, behaviors, interpersonal relationships, and cognitive function.

Independent Living

- This term refers to the use of transportation, money management, shopping, housekeeping, meal preparation, and the use of the community resources.
- Observe for clients' actual demands in their living situation, taking note of how well they can respond.

Mobility

- Evaluating a clients' mobility includes observing how they maneuver in their environment.
- The assessment includes observing how well clients ambulate, transfer, use assistive devices, and navigate stairs or obstacles (such as unleveled grounds).

Senses and Functions

- Assess the client for any physical deficits regarding muscle strength, range of motion, and balance. Since the majority of clients with AD are elderly, comorbid conditions can play a part in their debilitation.
- Determine whether and how the deficiencies interfere with their functional ability.

Self-Care

- Observe for the ability to complete personal care (dressing, feeding, personal hygiene, toileting, and sleeping patterns). Document any barriers clients encounter, especially with toileting.
- Focus on ways clients can maximize their independence.

See Module 3 for more lecture material.

Behaviors and Interpersonal Relationships

- Observe the client's relationships with others through the use of communication skills, affect, and emotional responses.
- The quality of each interaction should be monitored for the client's judgment and understanding.
- The client's response to frustration and conflict should also be observed.

Cognitive Function

- The client's perceptual-motor abilities, memory, and orientation should be noted.
- The caregiver should concentrate on the client's ability to overcome deficits.

Use all the components to help formulate an effective plan to assist the client. Ongoing evaluation is vital. Observe and report all the client's strengths and weakness to the supervisor. Staff and caregivers can assist each other by sharing perceived problems and highlighting any changes that need to be considered.

Insert agency's policy for reporting changes in the client's condition here.

Lecture Material for Slide 5-8

WANDERING

Wandering is one of the most common and life-threatening behaviors associated with AD and related disorders. According to the Alzheimer's Association, at least 60% of clients with dementia wander.

- Elopement and wandering are the most costly risk issues in long-term care. An elopement is a purposeful and frequently repeated attempt to leave the unit. Wandering is moving about the environment aimlessly and/or without a rational purpose or regard for personal safety. Both behaviors are dangerous.
- The confused and disoriented client may appear drunk or crazy to others who are not familiar with the disease. When clients become lost, strangers may try to avoid them, increasing the risk of injury.
- Not everyone with Alzheimer's disease wanders, but, for those who do, several precautions and practices must be part of the caregiver's daily routine.

Types of Wandering

Wandering is a manifestation of impaired brain function. Individuals wander for different reasons. Knowing the cause of the wandering behavior can help caregivers determine the reason, and find solutions to minimize the risks.

Searching

Searching is the act of looking for something. The client may be looking for a place or item from the present or the past.

Escaping

Escaping is the act of breaking free from confinement. The client may be trying to leave due to a perceived fear or threat.

Purposeful

Purposeful wandering is the act of achieving a desired goal. The client may be attempting to fulfill a previous responsibility such as cooking, getting ready for work, or tending to children (attempting to maintain previous roles).

Aimless

Aimless wandering consists of behaviors without purpose. The client may have underlying issues, which are unknown to caregivers or family. The act of wandering can be due to boredom, or the client may be using the action as a job.

REASONS FOR WANDERING

Lecture Material for Slide 5-9

All behaviors are forms of communication and have meaning. Wandering is no exception. Finding the reasons behind the wandering enables caregivers to limit the unwanted behavior.

Emotional

- Wandering may be viewed as a worthless act of time and energy to those without a cognitive impairment. To a client with dementia, wandering can act as a stress-reduction exercise, an expression of grief, or a coping mechanism.
- Wandering may be the by-product of a client searching for a deceased relative or spouse.
- The client may pace out of frustration. Think about how people pace when nervous.
- The client may be escaping from a perceived threat. (After the client hears screaming from the television, she begins to wander away from the noise.)

Recreational

- Many individuals have incorporated walking regimens into their daily routines. This goal does not disappear in clients with dementia. If the act of walking was a meaningful part of the daily routine prior to the disease process it, may still bring joy to them.
- All recreational activities should have a high success rate and require little decision-making skills.

Medical Causes

- Changes in clients' physical condition may cause changes in their behaviors. A physical exam should be conducted to rule out infections, injuries, pain, or reactions to medications.
- The client may wander due to an uncomfortable chair or article of clothing.
- Urinary tract infections are common in the elderly population. The client may be searching for the bathroom, due to the urgency and frequency of urination.

Nocturnal Wandering

- AD clients suffer from time disorientation and sleep disturbances.
- Clients in the beginning stages of AD awake at night and may be extremely confused, wanting to wander outside or act on a delusion.
- Many times a client awakens during the night and proceeds to get dressed and carry on daytime routines. Some take on preillness duties and prepare for the workday.
- Clients with sleep disturbances should remain active during the day. Naps and rest periods should be kept to a minimum. An exercise program should be incorporated into the daily routine to help them expel energy and cause fatigue.
- Maintaining the established nighttime rituals helps the client prepare for bedtime. Routines encourage security.

Lecture Material for Slides 5-10 and 5-11

Slide 5-10

During this portion of the lecture, the instructor should review the agency's elopement prevention program.

ELOPEMENT-PREVENTION PROGRAMS

An elopement-prevention program is a plan developed by the agency to prevent clients from wandering off units and sites. The plan encompasses all aspects of patient safety and rights.

- Assist the supervisor in identifying wandering-prone individuals upon admission by assessing whether clients have a risk for elopement. Determine whether they have a history of wandering by utilizing information from multiple sources: family members, physicians, or records of previous admissions.
- Report all observations to aid in the development of an elopement-prevention plan. Base the plan on the type and severity of risks associated with the individual's wandering behaviors. The plan should be client focused and continually updated and revised as necessary.

The warning signs for wandering include:

- Returning late from routine walks or drives.
- Expressing a desire to "go home," even when home.

- Attempting to return to previous roles (going to work, child care, homemaking, and such).
- Manifesting signs of restlessness, pacing, and other repetitive movements.

Slide 5-11

- Difficulty locating common spaces (the bathroom or bedroom).
- Looking for family and friends.
- Not completing tasks or activities.
- Appearing lost in their surroundings.

Reporting an Elopement

Insert the agency's policy regarding protocol on reporting an elopement.

- When a client has been returned safely after wandering or eloping, report the event to the supervisor following agency protocol. Report the occurrence even if the elopement was due to neglect or insubordination. Most of the elopements resulting in serious injuries or death were due to the lack of communication of previous elopements to all staff members.
- The incident should be communicated to all staff members on each shift.
- Documentation of the incident should include the risk of the client leaving again and strategies to reduce the risk of another occurrence.
- A staff member should keep the client under visual supervision at all times until interventions to reduce uncontrolled wandering are developed.
- Publications in the media and legal journals report that many institutions lack protocols governing the expectations of staff to report the incidence of elopement once a client is returned to the unit.

Lecture Material for Slide 5-12

● MANAGEMENT OF WANDERING

A well trained staff, in combination with a therapeutically supportive environment, can minimize the risk of wandering. The caregiver's role must be acknowledged as the first line of defense for the prevention of uncontrolled wandering and elopement incidents.

- The first tool when overseeing clients with Alzheimer's disease is flexibility. The second tool is creativity.
- The uniqueness of each person is forever changing and what worked today may not work tomorrow.
- Interventions are used to help maintain the goals of dementia care: safety, independence, and self-determination.

Ways to Reduce Wandering Behaviors

Caregivers must be creative when faced with the challenge of a client who wanders. A successful intervention is the discovery of what keeps the wanderer content today.

Providing Structured and Meaningful Activities

- Find activities to engage the dementia client. Persons who are occupied in a pleasant way do not get bored or frustrated. Boredom and frustration can cause wandering or other unwanted behaviors. Improving the self-esteem with successful activities only heightens clients' quality of life.

- Adapt activities to clients' changing capabilities and different moods. Providing structure gives AD clients security at the same time meeting the needs of their current circumstance.

- The key to a meaningful activity is keeping clients engaged in something interesting and important. Knowing their past occupations, hobbies, community interests, and the names of relatives can make any encounter meaningful. Enticing clients with a former interest or questions about their background can be a useful diversion.

- Uncontrolled events, such as an emergency or patterns of heightened activity, increase the opportunity for wandering. Changes of shift, the end of visiting hours, or unplanned events cause distractions; the staff may have needed to attend to different matters and lost sight of the client. The commotion causes overstimulation, intensifying wandering behaviors, and, because the caregiver is preoccupied by the event, the client has time to flee. For example, the well dressed senior can blend in with departing visitors, to be missed only after she has entered the unprotected environment.

- Inclement weather poses additional threats to the wandering client. Protocols should be in place during high-risk times to prevent such occurrences.

Insert agency's protocols for wandering during heightened activities.

Distracting the Individual

- When trying to distract an individual from wandering, use a creative method. Choose activities that can be easily completed to avoid frustration.

- The use of reminiscence helps the client recall happier times and reduces the stress causing the wandering.

- Engage the client in helping to complete a task, reinforcing his or her sense of usefulness.

- Design activities around the client's pre-illness days, whether on a professional or a personal level.

- Approach clients from the front, gently take hold of their hand, guide them to a safe area that is free of distractions, and initiate the activity. Use activities such as looking at newspapers, magazines, or photos.

Offer to play cards or ask them to sort the mail. Even encouraging them to pay the monthly bills by writing out pretend checks can quickly eliminate the need to wander.

Observation and Reporting

- Observation and reporting are important interventions when deterring uncontrolled wandering. The amount of restlessness, outbursts, and emotional responses should be included with all information reported. Any subtle change should be reported and not overlooked. Any changes are the precursors to potential problems.
- Observe the client for mood and behavioral changes. Does the client appear uncomfortable, bored, or craving additional personal contact?
- Observe the client for sensory overload. Is the environment loud and overwhelming? Excessive noise creates an information burden for the client.
- Observe clients for the use of visual or hearing aids. Any changes in their perception of information can trigger wandering. They could be fearful of the distorted images and wander as an escape. They may just be searching to find their glasses and become lost.
- Observe for changes in the daily routine or environment. The smallest modification in environment can create a significant behavioral change.

Exploring the Causes and Solutions for the Wandering Behavior

- Interventions should be multifaceted and geared as much as possible to the specific needs of the individual. If one technique fails, there should be other safeguards in place. Risk behaviors should be routinely reviewed to discover the strategies and safeguards that work best for the client.
- Find the who, what, where, and why of the wandering. Take note of the client's physical condition. Does the client exhibit signs of pain or discomfort? Are there any unexplained odors? Has there been a change in the medication regime?
- Evaluate the environment. Has there been a change in staffing or activities?
- Try to determine the type of wandering. The interventions should be based on meeting the unfulfilled need. Is the client searching for a lost item? Out of fear is the client trying to escape? Does the wandering have a purpose or does it appear to be aimless?

Safe Return Programs

Register the client in the Alzheimer's Association's Safe Return® program or other community return programs.

- The Alzheimer's Associations' Safe Return® program is a nationwide identification, support, and enrollment program providing assistance to persons with AD or other related dementias. Members receive a bracelet or necklace with their personal information. The program provides accessibility to law enforcement agencies and 24-hour expert guidance to help find missing cognitively impaired persons. (Alzheimer's Association)

- Safe Return® faxes local law enforcement with personal information about the missing individual. If a lost dementia client is not found within the first 24 hours, up to one-half of the victims will suffer serious harm or death. Safe Return has successfully found and returned 98% of the registered people with dementia who wandered and became lost. (Alzheimer's Association)

Insert agency's descriptions of its return programs and monitoring devices used at the facility.

Controlled Wandering

Wandering can be a stimulating and a therapeutic source of activity, exercise, and entertainment in a safe and controlled environment. Controlled wandering can contribute to a better night's sleep or an afternoon nap. Daytime wandering can deter sundowning and nocturnal wandering. Most importantly, wandering can allow a degree of independence within the controlled environment.

- Controlled wandering sets boundaries for the client to pace in a hazard-free zone. The area should include places to rest, handrails, and monitoring capabilities. Observe the client for fatigue, injury, or need for assistance.
- The path should be well lit and hazard free. A calm, quiet environment, free of extrinsic noises, can make this activity an enjoyable experience for the client.
- Wandering paths offer the benefit of repeated trips along the same path, limiting the area that needs to be carefully safety proofed and constantly supervised. The client should not be able to wander into an unsecured area or leave the unit altogether.
- Walking groups can be established to improve socialization.

Things to Know

- To prevent clients from utilizing an area, use a dark colored mat in front of the area, it may be perceived as a hole or a place to avoid.
- Install warning bells or monitoring devices that signal when a door is opened.
- Label all doors, using signs or symbols defining the space.
- Camouflage doors by painting them the same color as the walls.
- Observe and report wandering behaviors to the supervisor.
- Use child safety locks and adaptive door handles.

Lecture Material for Slides 5-13 and 5-14

Slide 5-13

FALL PREVENTION

Falls are common with the elderly population, but particularly those with Alzheimer's disease. Research has found a correlation between AD and a higher incidences in falls. As the brain deteriorates, the dementia client experiences problems with mobility. As with completing a successful activity, the client needs a level of cognitive functioning to walk, climb stairs, avoid barriers, or use durable medical equipment (DME).

Reasons for Falls

Observing the client's abilities and evaluating risk factors can assist with maintaining safety and preventing falls.

Age-Related Changes Contributing to Falls

- Clients may have problems understanding the spoken word, leading to more disorientation. Hearing loss among the elderly can be related to the thinning of the membrane and calcification of the small bones in the middle ear or atrophic changes in the ear itself. The progression of hearing loss may result in the client's having distorted speech.

- In normal aging, changes in the lens of the eye decrease vision. Pastel colors are less distinguishable; primary colors are better seen. The person's ability to adapt from light to darkness (adaptation) also decreases. The aging person needs more light to see. Changes in the lens of the eye cause the client to experience more glare in their vision. The damage to the occipital lobe of the brain due to plaque formation exacerbates the visual problems for the AD client. Any of these distortions can contribute to the client's risks of falls. The aging process may impact the delusional images seen by the dementia client.

- The age-related changes in the arterial walls cause orthostatic hypotension, causing dizziness and lightheadedness.

- A decrease in muscle cells (muscle mass) and a reduction in the blood supply to the muscles occur with aging. As a result, muscles respond more slowly to stimuli and tire easily. Deterioration of the joints causes a decrease in range of motion.

Cognitive Changes

- Individuals with Alzheimer's disease react more slowly than normal, making it more difficult for them to regain their balance. The series of tasks necessary to use the arms to protect the body when falling is too complex for the failing brain.

- Visual agnosia is the lost ability to identify what is being seen.

- The person's inability to perceive direction, along with the uncertainty in self-positioning and coordinated movements, hinders the client's ability to distinguish between self and objects. (The client may fall just by leaning when sitting on the toilet.)

- During the course of the disease, clients lose the ability to have coordinated movements (ataxia). The client's unsteady gait causes difficulties with all activities of daily living. The reason for the unsteadiness is unknown and usually appears after memory and language disturbances are apparent.

- Persons with AD may not be able to gauge the height of steps, curbs, and door thresholds accurately.
- Dementia clients may fall when trying to avoid an imagined obstacle, protecting themselves from a perceived stranger, or defending personal space.
- AD clients take more risk due to their impaired judgment. They may attempt to climb on the edge of a chair to reach for something, even if doing so is not safe.

Fall Prevention Program

Review agency's fall prevention policy here.

Things to Know

- All employees can prevent falls.
- All clients are at risk for falls, regardless of age.
- Observe clients for their need for assistance when ambulating, standing, changing positions.
- Observe for adverse reactions and side effects of medications.
- Control environmental risk factors: wet floors, lighting, and scatter rugs.
- Remind the client to use all corrective devices (eyeglasses, hearing aids) and DME (eg, a cane or walker). Encourage the use of grab bars and handrails.
- Maintain clutter-free pathways.
- Remove any conditions that may trigger the client to fall. For example, falls can occur when clients attempt to obtain out of reach items.
- Reinforce a toileting schedule when appropriate.
- Limit the use of restraints.
- Encourage proper footwear.
- Advocate exercise to increase strength and muscle tone.
- Report all falls to the supervisor.

CHOOSING AN ACTIVITY

As stressed throughout the module, all activities should be selected based on the client's individuality and abilities. The task should always be challenging, intellectually stimulating, and successful.

- Provide positive reinforcement throughout the activity but do not overpraise.

- Once clients have successfully achieved an activity, incorporate it into their routine. Do not have them perform the task for extended periods of time; the activity will become meaningless to them and appear as "busy work."

Montessori Principles

With Montessori education, learning occurs in a helpful environment characterized by friendly interaction and peer teaching. Dr. Cameron J. Camp, PhD (1999) adapted the principles of Montessori to be used with clients with dementia. The following summarizes his approach:

- Use real-life materials whenever possible.
- Advance from the simple to the complex.
- Proceed from the concrete to the abstract.
- Arrange materials from the largest to the smallest and from the most to the least.
- Allow learning to progress from observation, recognition, then demonstration.
- Practice each component of the activities one at a time.
- Minimize the risk of failure and maximize the chance of success by choosing activities that are appropriate for the individual.
- Use slow and deliberate movements when demonstrating an activity. Move at the client's pace.
- Make the materials and activity self-correcting.
- Have the client make something that can be used.
- Adapt the environment to the person's needs (eg, the height of the table).
- Encourage the client to select the activity whenever possible.
- Accommodate for any physical limitations (eg, eyeglasses, large print books).

Montessori principles can also aid in developing alterations in the complexity of an activity while still providing meaning and purpose. Adjusting the activity using different tasks with the same level of complexity is called horizontal programming. Changing the level of complexity of an existing activity is called vertical programming.

Audience Interaction for Slide 5-15

Ask the audience to provide examples of horizontal and vertical programming of a meaningful task, such as watering plants with a pitcher. Possible responses are:

- For horizontal programming: pouring cream into coffee or pouring water into glasses.
- For vertical programming: using a small cup of water instead of a pitcher to water the plants or administering plant fertilizer with an eyedropper.

Features of a Successful Activity

- Keep the activity short and simple, with few verbal instructions. Always take advantage of the client's previous skills.
- The optimum time for an activity is between 20 and 30 minutes. In the latter part of the disease, the length of client's participation may last for five to 10 minutes.
- Group activities should be limited to four to 10 participants. The group size is determined by the client's level of functioning.
- Use distraction if clients become upset. Discontinue the current activity and guide them toward a more appropriate task.
- Be creative if the chosen activity does not work. Flexibility is essential when caring for a client with dementia.
- The level of the activity should be adultlike. The task can be simplified for the client's ability but should remain purposeful. As the client's condition declines, the use of children's picture books and games may be appropriate.
- Schedule activities to accommodate fluctuations in the client's energy levels. Using a relaxing activity, such as listening to music, is more appropriate for evening hours than dancing, for example.

Examples of Activities for the Dementia Client

The following sample activities can be incorporated into the client's daily routine. The primary goal of any activity is for the client to experience the activity.

Reminiscence

Using reminiscence as the focus of an activity can help validate the client's life accomplishments. Recalling the past can be used during any stage of the disease.

Reminiscing activities can include:

- Story telling.
- Making a memory book or box.
- Reviewing old photos.
- Watching home movies.
- Reading old newspaper articles or watching movies from the client's era.
- Listening to music from the past.

Exercise

Adequate exercise relieves feelings of tension and anxiety. Incorporating physical exercise in the client's routine promotes fatigue and better rest periods.

Exercising can include:
- Walking.
- Active games (passing the ball, bowling, shuffleboard).
- Household chores (setting the table, dusting, raking leaves, mopping the floor, beating eggs).
- Stretching.
- Chair exercises.
- Dancing.

Crafts

Crafts are suitable only for persons who have a long enough attention span to complete the work. The activities need to be purposeful and adultlike, not just busywork. Select projects that appeal to the client's interest and skill level.

Crafting can include:
- Making a collage.
- Making a gift for family or friends.
- Stringing beads.
- Drawing.

Socializing

As stated earlier, all human beings have a basic need to be loved, to be useful, and to express feelings. Socialization allows the client to be part of a nurturing relationship. Communication skills are at the heart of any social interaction. Given the right support, clients with dementia are still capable of having a brief and meaningful conversation.

Socializing activities include:
- Support groups.
- Coffee breaks and mealtimes.
- Field trips.
- Viewing family photos.
- Theme discussions (talking about the war, fashions, movies, etc.).
- Assistance with personal care.

Meal Preparation

Meal preparation and cooking involve all the senses: sight, sound, smells, touch, and taste. Cooking allows the client to enjoy the outcome of the activity.

Activities for meal preparation can include:
- Adding ingredients to the bowl.
- Beating eggs.

- Decorating cookies and cakes.
- Filling sugar and creamer bowls.
- Filling water glasses at mealtime.
- Washing fruits and vegetables.

Fragrances and Scents

Sensory memory is the retention of actual sensory images. Clients with profound cognitive loss can still find joy in the smell of roses.

Fragrance and scent activities include:

- Making scented sachets.
- Smelling flowers or herbs.
- Smelling fragrant woods (eg, cedar, redwood).
- Enjoying the aromas of foods.
- Using fragrant hand lotion.
- Smelling the scent of freshly cut grass.

Family Visits

As the disease progresses, family members may find it difficult to "connect" with their loved ones. By making use of the abilities that persist, the family can continue to connect with and bring joy to their relative. Focus on stimulating the lifetime experiences of the client. Coach the family on ways to make visits more meaningful.

Family can make visits more meaningful by:

- Bringing a favorite treat.
- Sharing "your day."
- Talking about lifetime accomplishments.
- Having a music visit.
- Completing a project together.
- Doing "what you did together" (eg, watching a favorite show, manicures, hobbies).

SUMMING UP

Alzheimer's disease erodes a person's cognitive functioning. Everyday activities, which come natural to most, become laborious for the dementia client. Changes in role and the lack of successful activities wear down the self-esteem of the individual. The repeated failure of daily activities creates more boundaries and can lead to challenging behaviors.

When planning activities, include responsibilities from the individual's previous stages of life. The activities that make up a client's day provide a sense of usefulness, pleasure, and success. Activities should enrich the client's life. The center point of dementia care should be maximizing independence while focusing on strengths and abilities.

Wandering occurs for many reasons and imposes many dangers for those with Alzheimer's disease. Various cognitive deficiencies and patterns of wandering are common in both long-term care and assisted living facilities. The greater the degree of the client's cognitive impairment, the greater the risk is for wandering and elopement behavior. Observation, education, and strategies help manage wandering.

Instructor's Version with Answers to Handout 5-2

● REAL-LIFE SCENARIO

A Day in the Life of Pat

Pat has always been very organized. All family photos and papers were neatly filed and stacked in the proper cabinet. As a former schoolteacher, Pat is accustomed to following plans to achieve the desired outcome. Recently, Pat has been arriving late for meals and is often not dressed appropriately.

1. In terms of Zgola's functional evaluation, in which components does Pat exhibit weaknesses?

   Based on the information provided, Pat's limitations, according to Zgola's functional evaluation, should be assessed using the seven Ws and evaluated in the following areas:

   - *Independent living: The demands of Pat's living situation may be greater than current abilities. Pat is having difficulty arriving on time for meals.*
   - *Mobility: Pat's ability to maneuver through the living space to the dining hall may have too many obstacles to overcome and may be greater than current abilities.*
   - *Senses and functions: A physical assessment should determine if Pat's inability to dress appropriately is due to physical deficits regarding muscle strength, range of motion, or balance.*
   - *Self-care: Pat's inappropriate attire leads to questions regarding the ability to complete personal care.*
   - *Behaviors and interpersonal relationships: Pat may be embarrassed by weakened communications skills and arrives late to avoid socialization with other residents.*
   - *Cognitive function: The intellectual functions of memory, abstract thinking, organization, perception, attention span, and judgment may be affecting Pat's success in activities and should be evaluated.*

2. List possible reasons for Pat's wandering behavior.

   Wandering is a behavior, which has meaning. The possible reasons for wandering include emotional, recreational, medical, or time disorientation.

3. List activities that would be appropriate for Pat. Explore horizontal and vertical programming for each example given.

   Since Pat relished organization, design activities with structure and pattern. Examples are making a photo album or organizing paperwork, concentrating on Pat's strengths and weaknesses.

   Horizontal programming would involve stuffing letters into envelopes or placing papers into folders. Vertical programming would involve looking at photo albums or helping assemble the daily calendar of events.

GROUP ACTIVITY

● PURPOSE OF THE ACTIVITY

The purpose of this activity is to review the necessary cognitive resources required for the completion of a successful activity. The following can be completed as a class, in small groups, or individually.

Ask the audience to describe the cognitive resources needed to make a bed. Answers should comprise the need to understand the verbal command (language skills) and remembering what the task is to complete (memory). Include the following in the discussion:

- Conceptualizing the term "making the bed," not the literal meaning of manufacturing a bed (abstract thought).
- Organizing the task in sequence: smoothing out the flat sheet, followed by the blankets, repositioning the pillows, fixing the comforter, and so on (organization).
- Completing each task in the appropriate sequence without becoming distracted (attention).
- Utilizing the sense of touch and sight (perception).
- Making decisions when encountering a problem. What to do if the sheet is caught on the bed frame (judgment).
- Evaluating the quality of the work completed (judgment).

Name _____ Date _____

Program/Course _____ Instructor's Name _____

Recreation Activities Pre- and Post-Test

1. What can activities do for a person?
    a. Activities can fulfill psychosocial needs.
    b. Activities provide the physical stress needed for normal cell growth.
    c. Activities define a person.
    d. All of the above.

2. Define sensory memory.
    a. Sensory memory is the retention of actual sensory images in the sensory area of the brain.
    b. Sensory memory refers to the accumulation of facts and experiences over a lifetime.
    c. Sensory memory measures the ability of the client to remember events occurring the same day.
    d. Sensory memory is learned by repetitive movements.

3. Wandering is one of the most common and life-threatening behaviors associated with AD. According to the Alzheimer's Association, what percentage of dementia clients wander?
    a. 75%
    b. 60%
    c. 23%
    d. 18%

4. A dementia client may wander because he or she is:
    a. Looking for something.
    b. Trying to leave the area due to fear.
    c. Attempting to fulfill previous responsibilities.
    d. All of the above.

5. When formulating an activity plan for a client with dementia, the primary goal should be the client's:
    a. Physical health and behavioral symptoms.
    b. Experience of the activity.
    c. Orientation and awareness of the environment.
    d. Language and communication skills.

Handout **5-1**

A Day in the Life of Pat: A Real-Life Scenario

Pat has always been very organized. All family photos and papers were neatly filed and stacked in the proper cabinet. As a former schoolteacher, Pat is accustomed to following plans to achieve the desired outcome. Recently, Pat has been arriving late for meals and is often not dressed appropriately.

1. In terms of Zgola's functional evaluation, in which components does Pat exhibit weaknesses?

2. List possible reasons for Pat's wandering behavior.

3. List activities that would be appropriate for Pat. Explore horizontal and vertical programming for each example given.

MODULE 5 RECREATION AND ACTIVITIES

Transparency Master **5-1**

Purposeful Activities Will:

- **Enhance feelings of self-worth**
- **Create enjoyment**
- **Promote general health**
- **Preserve memory**
- **Maintain communication skills**
- **Improve personal relationships**

Purposeful Activities Will: (*cont.*)

- **Promote family interactions**
- **Increase muscle strength**
- **Reduce nervous tension**
- **Decrease pacing/ restlessness/wandering**
- **Increase nighttime sleep**

Requirements for a Successful Activity

- Language skills
- Memory
- Abstract thought
- Organization skills
- Perception
- Attention span
- Judgment

Making an Activity Successful

- **Promote strengths**
- **Maintain goals**
- **Observation and reporting**

Zgola's 7 W's of a Functional Evaluation

- **W**hat can the client do?
- **W**hat does the client do?
- Ho**w** does he or she do it?
- **W**hich parts of the task is the client unable to do? and **W**hy?
- **W**here or **w**hen does he or she perform best?

Components of a Functional Evaluation

- Independent living
- Mobility
- Senses and functions
- Self-care
- Behaviors and interpersonal relationships
- Cognitive function

Types of Wandering

- **Searching**
- **Escaping**
- **Purposeful**
- **Aimless**

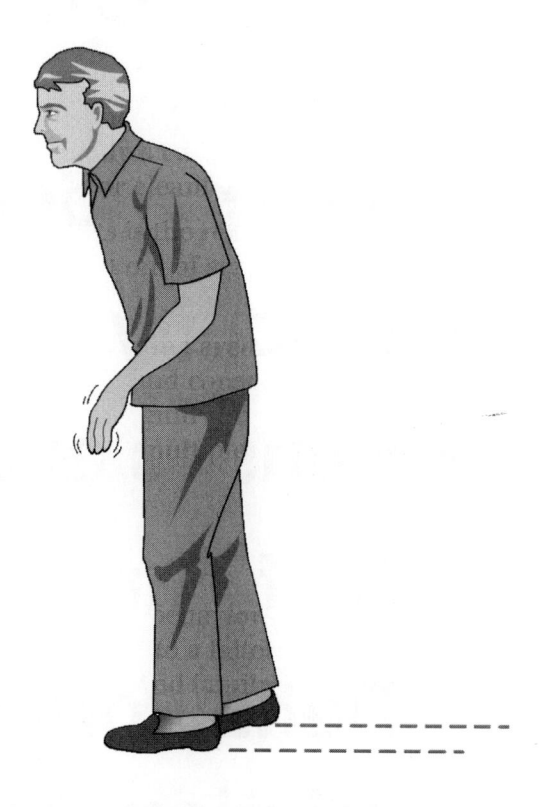

Reasons for Wandering

- **Emotional**
- **Recreational**
- **Medical**
- **Nocturnal**

Warning Signs for Wandering

- **Returning late from routine walks or drives**
- **Expressing a desire to "go home"**
- **Returning to previous roles**
- **Symptoms of restlessness**

Warning Signs for Wandering (cont.)

- **Difficulties locating common spaces**
- **Looking for family or friends**
- **Not completing tasks**
- **Appearing lost**

Ways to Reduce Wandering Behaviors

- **Structured and meaningful activities**
- **Distraction**
- **Observation and reporting**
- **Explore causes and solutions**

Fall Prevention

- Everyone can prevent falls
- Every person is at risk
- Observe abilities
- Monitor medication side effects
- Reduce environmental risks
- Reinforce use of corrective devices

Fall Prevention (cont.)

- **Maintain clutter free pathways**
- **Remove triggers**
- **Reinforce toileting schedules**
- **Limit restraints**
- **Encourage proper footwear**
- **Advocate exercise**
- **Report all falls**

Features of a Successful Activity

- **Simplicity**
- **Time-frame**
- **Distractibility**
- **Creativity**
- **Purposeful and adult like**
- **Scheduling**

Module 6
Common Medical Problems

Goal
To better understand the normal aging process and medical problems associated with dementia.

Objectives
After the completion of the presentation, students will be able to:

- Describe the normal aging process.
- Describe the difference between normal aging and dementia.
- Name four common medical conditions associated with dementia.
- List what is included in a pain assessment.
- Explain the symptoms observed in the late stage of Alzheimer's disease.
- Describe the general components of end-of-life care for a dementia client.

Lecture Material for Slide 6-1

GENERAL INFORMATION/OVERVIEW

During the course of AD, clients may develop additional medical conditions that impact their quality of life and contribute to their death. The stage of dementia and the medical conditions should both be considered when developing a treatment plan.

The following statistics are from *The State of Aging and Health in America* (Merck, 2004):

- For persons born in 1900 the life expectancy was 47 years, compared to 2001 when the life expectancy was 77 years. The consequences of a greater life expectancy are chronic illnesses and degenerative diseases. One in ten persons over the age of 65 is estimated to have Alzheimer's disease, and nearly one half of people over the age of 85 are afflicted with this disease.

- Currently, at least 80% of older Americans are living with at least one chronic condition, and 50% have at least two.

- Since dementia usually occurs in the second half of life, primarily over the age of 65, seniors develop more symptoms of dementia, as well as other chronic illnesses, than those of a younger age.

- The average person over the age of 75 has three chronic conditions and uses five prescription drugs.

Lecture Material for Slide 6-2 and Handout 6-2

Review Handout 6-2 with the lecture material.

THE NORMAL AGING PROCESS

The process of normal aging, in the absence of disease, is accompanied by vast changes. Aging affects all body systems to varying degrees among individuals. Genetics and long-term lifestyle factors impact the aging process.

Anatomical and physiological changes attributed to aging, may alter the elderly person's response to illness. Normal age-associated changes must be differentiated from pathological processes to develop appropriate interventions. Aging and illness can affect the presentation of symptoms, the response to treatment, and outcomes.

Theory on Aging

- The by-product of the oxygen used by the body (free radicals) may cause normal age-associated changes. Free radicals have lost one electron and seek to stabilize themselves by stealing an electron from a nearby molecule. The free radicals are not choosy about where they get their electrons and readily attach to and damage healthy cells.

- The body has a natural defense against the free radicals called antioxidants. These chemicals limit the activity of the free radicals

and repair the damage. The aging client's cells generate fewer or less efficient antioxidants.
- The theory of damage related to free radicals may explain why many diseases (heart disease, cancer, cataracts) become more common with age.

Skin, Nails, and Hair (Integumentary System)
- Changes in appearance, especially the skin, are the most obvious signs of aging. An increase in the amount of visible wrinkles is due to the reduction of elastin in the skin, a decrease in fat under the skin, and decreased circulation. Different ethnic groups have fewer wrinkles due to the natural oils in the skin. Gravity causes the loose skin to hang at the jaw and neck.
- Pigment changes of the skin (age spots) are more noticeable in the older adult. The skin has less protection as a result of the reduction of underlying fat. Capillaries are more visible, and the skin has an increased risk of bruising and tearing. The skin may resemble plastic wrap or cellophane. The decreased fat and muscle tone of the feet can affect ambulation.
- The thinned fat layer also reduces the covering of joints and bony prominences (eg, wrist bone), increasing the risk for pressure ulcers and injuries. A decrease in sensation may also occur, increasing the risk for injury.
- Skin has a decrease in elasticity, turgor, and wound healing. Skin is dryer and paler in appearance than when younger.
- The aging person perspires less due to the reduction in sweat and sebaceous glands, resulting in a reduction of body temperature maintenance.
- Nails become thick, brittle, yellow, and split due to decreased circulation. Chronic conditions of diabetes and heart disease compound these effects. Hair becomes finer. The loss of hair in men is due to the decrease in the hormone testosterone. The increase in facial hair on women is due to the decrease in the hormone estrogen.
- Gray hair is caused by a decrease in melanocytes.

Vision
- Changes in the lens of the eye cause a decrease in vision. Pastel colors are less distinguishable, and primary colors are better seen.
- The person's ability to adapt from light to darkness (adaptation) also decreases. The aging person needs more light to see. Changes in the lens of the eye cause clients to experience more glare in their vision.
- Older adults experience a decrease in night vision and an alteration in depth perception.

- Vitreous floaters (floating matter seen by the eyes) are more common among the aging.
- Cataracts (the clouding of the lens) are an abnormal progressive condition of the lens of the eye characterized by the loss of transparency. A white film can be observed over the lens and iris. The loss of transparency reduces eyesight.
- Glaucoma is a disease of the eye caused by an increase in intraocular pressure. A gradual loss of peripheral vision occurs over time, resulting in tunnel vision. Eye drops and medications are prescribed to treat the condition.
- Presbyopia is the inability to see objects up close and requires corrective lenses. The client may not be able to read a medication bottle.
- Age-related macular degeneration is the formation of spots on the retina, making vision difficult.

Auditory System

- Hearing loss can be associated with the thinning of the membrane, calcification of the small bones in the middle ear, or atrophic changes in the ear itself.
- Presbycusis is the most common cause of hearing loss in this age group, resulting in the inability to hear high-frequency sounds.
- Progressive hearing loss may cause the client to develop distorted speech. When environmental noise interferes with poorly articulated speech, the client may have additional problems comprehending the conversation. Hearing problems may limit a person's socialization and can be a safety hazard (eg, not hearing the fire alarm).
- Dry earwax (cerumen), with the risk of impaction, ringing in the ears (tinnitus), and equilibrium balance deficits, are also associated with aging.

Smell (Olfactory System)

- The aging process causes a decrease in the function of cranial nerves. The sense of smell lessens with age due to the decrease in the olfactory nerves.
- Smell can have an impact on a client's appetite.
- The loss of smell may inhibit the client from smelling gas or smoke.

Oral Cavity

- Taste perceptions, such as sweet, salty, sour, and bitter, are altered with aging. Food preferences may change accordingly.
- Loose, missing teeth, poorly fitting dentures, or gum disorders are commonly associated with aging. The client may have difficulty chewing food.
- The aging client may experience a dry mouth due to the decrease in saliva and atrophy of the oral mucosa.

Respiratory System

- Degenerative changes limit the chest wall expansion during the respiratory cycle, making breathing more difficult. The breaths are not as deep as they were when the client was younger.
- Thorax changes decrease the ability to breath and cough deeply, leading to a higher incidence of infection or pneumonia.
- A decrease in the number of alveoli (the area for the exchange of oxygen and carbon dioxide) results in a decrease in oxygen saturation. Shortness of breath (dyspnea) upon exertion may be observed.

Circulatory System

- Aging causes a decreased efficiency in the heart muscle. An aging heart can still be a healthy heart.
- The heart rate is lower than that of a younger adult. The conduction system of the heart, which controls heart rate, is disrupted; abnormal heart rhythms (dysrhythmias) are common.
- After exercise or other cardiovascular activity, the older adult's heart rate takes longer to return to normal.
- With age, veins and arteries accumulate calcium deposits and have changes in blood vessel elasticity. The calcium deposits increase peripheral resistance on the vessels, in turn causing an increase in the systolic and diastolic blood pressure values. Changes in blood pressure, when clients stand up quickly (orthostatic hypotension), can make them feel lightheaded or dizzy.
- Cardiovascular disease is the most common medical problem in the elderly. Conditions include congestive heart disease, myocardial infarctions (heart attack), and high blood pressure (hypertension).
- Edema of the lower extremities is the result of poor coronary function. Slow healing sores (stasis ulcers) can develop and are produced by the pooling of blood from leaky valves in the veins.

Musculoskeletal System

- Changes in the musculoskeletal system vary greatly among individuals. Healthy eating, routine exercise, and the predisposition to certain conditions can impact musculoskeletal function.
- Decreased muscle strength and agility, along with slowed deep tendon reflexes and reaction times, are due to, the alteration in muscle mass (muscle cells) and the reduction in blood supply to the muscles.
- A decrease in mineral absorption results in brittle bones. Narrowed intervertebral disks may lead to height loss (kyphosis) of one to four inches.
- Joint stiffness with decreased mobility leads to an increase risk of injury. Arthritis, joint subluxation, crackling or grating under the skin (crepitus), and pain on range of motion are frequent complaints of the senior client. Gait and balance instability are also common.

- A decrease in strength is related to the activity level of the client or the disease process. If the client has a sedentary lifestyle, the muscles become weaker. Aging does not cause weak muscles.

Gastrointestinal System

- Aging causes a decrease in the production of saliva and gastric juices during the digestive process. The reduction of digestive enzymes causes indigestion or heartburn. The client experiences a greater number of food intolerances.
- Changes in weight can result with aging. Daily energy requirements for the aging body are reduced. The caloric intake also needs to be reduced to prevent unwanted weight gain.
- A diminished gag reflex and food remaining in the esophagus longer may contribute to the aspiration (the inhalation of regurgitated gastric contents into the pulmonary system) of vomitus.
- Constipation is due to a slower rate of peristalsis. A frequent problem among the elderly causing them to fixate on bowel movements.

Immune System

- The body's defense system becomes less effective with age, decreasing the ability to fight infection.
- With the aging process comes an increase in the number of autoantibodies. The rise in the number of autoantibodies increases the risk of developing an autoimmune disease.

Endocrine System

- Pancreas and thyroid gland hormones (insulin, T3, T4) are diminished in the healthy aging client.
- With advanced age, the incidence of diabetes increases. Diabetes is a condition affecting the metabolism of sugar.
- Hypothyroidism is a condition caused by a decrease of the thyroid hormone, which is responsible for controlling metabolism. The client may experience thinning hair, constipation, and a lack of energy. Symptoms of low thyroid hormones are very similar to normal occurrences in the aging and may be overlooked as a diagnosis.
- Hormone levels of estrogen, progesterone, and testosterone are reduced.
- Changes in bone mineral density lead to the risk of osteoporosis and fractures. Osteoporosis causes the bones to lose density by forming voids inside the bone (think of the holes in Swiss cheese). Bones become more brittle and are easily broken. The weakening of the bones cause fractures, falls, and problems with balance.
- Alterations in the hormone levels produce changes in body composition with increased fat, decreased muscle, and reduced bone mass, resulting in a decrease in strength and function.

Urinary System

- The risk of renal complications with comorbid conditions accelerates with age. The elderly population is more susceptible to acute ischemic renal failure.
- A weakened bladder is caused by loss of muscle mass. The bladder cannot expand and contract as effectively, resulting in urinary retention or incontinence.
- The kidneys are reduced in size. Decreased blood flow to the kidneys reduces the filtration rate; thus urine is less concentrated.
- Residual urine in the bladder causes a urinary tract infection (UTI). Limited fluid intake also impacts the risk of a UTI. Urinary retention leads to infection and perforation of the bladder.
- Alteration in kidney filtration can lead to medication toxicity. Adverse side effects can become life threatening.
- In males, the incidence of urinary hesitancy, dribbling, frequency, and incontinence increases. The prostate gland enlarges (benign prostate hypertrophy [BPH]), causing difficulty with urination. Urinating during the night (nocturia) is the result of the decreased ability to hold urine and/or the enlargement of the prostate. Nocturia may contribute to falls and decreased sleep.
- In females, there is an increased risk for atrophic vaginitis, urethritis, vaginal stenosis, and vaginal/uterine prolapse. A prolapsed bladder may alarm a client when the bladder can be felt or palpated in the vaginal opening. This condition, which is benign, can inhibit a person's ability to fully empty the bladder.

Reproductive System

- The need for sexual intimacy and relationships does not disappear with age. The aging client is capable of having sexual intercourse. A decline in sexual energy is, however, noted.
- Changes in the cells of the female reproductive system and breast occur as estrogen levels decline. Menopause occurs between the ages of 45 and 60.
- Men experience a decline in the production of testosterone.
- The risk of prostate cancer rises with increased age. Impotency (erectile dysfunction, ED) in men can become a problem.
- Female clients may experience common menopause symptoms hot flashes, vaginal dryness, and mood swings. The incidence of breast cancer increases with age.

Nervous System

- The healthy aging adult experiences slowed thought processes, responses to stimuli, and reflexes. In the absence of disease, the aging process *does not* decrease intelligence.

- As the nervous system ages, degeneration in the neuron pathways produces changes in balance, gait, and coordinated movements (ischemic paresthesia).
- A decreased ability to respond to multiple stimuli and multitasking may be observed. Some short-term memory loss is expected.
- The elderly population has an increased threshold for light touch and pain sensation.
- The leading cause of disability in elderly aging is related to neurological impairments: Parkinson's disease, strokes, and Alzheimer's disease.

Lecture Material for Handout 6-3 (no slide)

NORMAL AGING AND DEMENTIA

Forgetting events, a person's name, or where items have been placed does not imply a diagnosis of Alzheimer's disease. "Senior moments," as they have been called, are a by-product of life and hectic schedules. With age, these moments may seem to happen more frequently. The normal aging process causes symptoms that, at times, may be mistaken for dementia. The following is a comparison of the differences between normal aging and dementia.

Normal Cognitive Changes with Aging

In the absence of disease, an aging person:

- Maintains ADL.
- Experiences intermittent memory loss, but retains pertinent details.
- Is more concerned with the memory loss than friends and family.
- Has no memory loss of recent events or affairs.
- Has unimpaired communications skills (despite occasional trouble with word searching).
- Demonstrates unaltered interpersonal skills.
- May momentarily forget directions to familiar areas but does not get lost.
- Has the ability to operate common appliances (even if he or she is unwilling to learn how to operate new devices or technology).
- Has cognitive functioning that is evaluated within normal limits.

Cognitive Changes with Dementia

A person with dementia:

- Needs assistance with all ADLs.
- Admits to memory loss only after being confronted and cannot supply details of the situation.
- Shows less concern about the memory loss than family and friends.
- Inability to remember recent events.

- Experiences problems with conversations (such as word searching difficulties, frequent pauses in dialogue, and word substitutions).
- Exhibits inappropriate social behaviors and is less interested in social events.
- Forgets directions and gets lost in familiar surroundings, sometimes taking hours to get home.
- Cannot operate common appliances or learn how to use new devices or technology.
- Has cognitive functioning evaluated below normal limits.

Things to Know

- Establish a baseline for the client and take a virtual snapshot photo. Compare the client's progress to the original observation. Include the client's cognitive abilities, memory, and communication skills.
- Report all symptoms and characteristic changes to the supervisor.
- Never assume that a new behavior or symptom is a normal part of aging.

Lecture Material for Slide 6-3

COMMON MEDICAL PROBLEMS

Clients with dementia may suffer from comorbid conditions. Late-stage dementia clients may die from these secondary illnesses, not from the Alzheimer's disease. Residing in a long-term care facility predisposes clients to various illnesses resulting from feeding problems and sedentary lifestyles. Conditions range from minor inconveniences to serious debilitating medical ailments. Dementia clients' altered cognition hinders their ability to verbalize discomfort. Caregivers may feel the dementia is worsening, only to realize that an underlying medical problem exists. When the medical problem is treated and resolved, the client's cognition may return to the recent baseline. Routinely performing a head-to-toe assessment can minimize such alterations.

Signs of Body System Changes

- Changes in behavior
- Increased agitation
- Nausea or vomiting
- Diarrhea
- Skin changes
- Coughing
- Respiratory congestion
- Increased lethargy
- Changes in gait
- Swelling of any extremity

Dehydration

Dehydration is a serious condition resulting from excessive fluid loss, occurring when fluid output exceeds fluid intake. Detailed lecture material on dehydration is presented later in the module.

Unreported Injuries

The elderly are at an increased risk of falls. Alteration in coordination and balance due to neuron death increases dementia clients' risk of injury. Clients may not report an incident due to altered judgment, even with a sustained injury. They may be unable to express their discomfort. Mood changes are often the first sign of an injury or pain.
Routinely monitor clients for:

- Bodily bruises, especially on the back, arm, knees, and legs.
- Blisters on the feet.
- Skin breakdown or skin shearing.
- Swelling of the feet and hands.
- Bumps on the head.
- Sores in the mouth.

Infections

An infection is a condition in which the body or a section of the body is invaded by a pathogen, causing serious complications. Additional lecture material will be furnished later in the module, exploring other infectious illnesses affecting the elderly.

Pneumonia

Pneumonia is an inflammation of the lungs caused by infectious organisms. Pneumonia is a significant health problem in the elderly and the fourth leading cause of death. Often the elderly develop pneumonia following a prolonged serious illness. Silent aspiration, oropharyngeal colonization from poor oral hygiene, abnormal swallowing, and decreased ambulation are predisposing factors for pneumonia in the elderly. *Streptococcus pneumonae* is the most common cause of bacterial pneumonia. The bacteria can multiply rapidly and cause damage even in the healthy. Those with a compromised immune system are at greater risk.

Risks for Developing Pneumonia

- Advanced age
- Influenza
- Comorbid conditions
- Chronic obstructive pulmonary disease (COPD)
- Diabetes
- Congestive heart failure (CHF)

Clinical Symptoms of Pneumonia
- Fever
- Chills
- Productive cough
- Acute confusion
- Difficulty breathing (tachypnea)
- Rapid heart rate (tachycardia)

Constipation

Constipation is the difficulty in passing stool and the passing of hard, dry stool. Peristalsis is slowed in the elderly, making them prone to constipation. Dementia clients may be unaware of the last time they had a bowel movement. They may be experiencing abdominal discomfort, but are unaware of its cause. Observe the client for abdominal distention and straining when passing stool. The risk of bowel impaction increases with chronic constipation. Monitor and report the frequency of all bowel movements.

Fecal Impaction

Fecal impaction is a collection of hardened fecal material in the rectum or sigmoid colon. Prolonged constipation causes additional water to be reabsorbed in the rectum, and the stool becomes harder and dryer. In this instance the stool needs to be manually removed.

Signs of Fecal Impaction
- Complaints of abdominal pain
- Complaints of rectal pain
- Nausea
- Lack of appetite
- Excessive flatulence
- Bloating
- Frequent urination
- Inability to empty the bladder
- Urge to have a bowel movement
- Liquid stool seeping around the obstruction
- Mental confusion in extreme cases

Complications from Prolonged Immobility

During the course of AD, clients experience a decline in their ability to move independently. End-stage Alzheimer's renders clients unable to speak, to respond to their environment, and ultimately to move. Prolonged immobility affects all body systems.

- Prolonged immobility increases the risk of pulmonary complications. A decrease in lung expansion and an increase in fluid accumulation cause respiratory tract infections and pneumonia.

- Slowed blood flow (venous stasis) increases the threat of a blood clot (thrombus) or a traveling blood clot (embolus). Changes in circulation cause swelling (edema) of the extremities.

- With reduced movement, muscles become weak and diminish in size and strength (atrophy). Contractures or deformities occur, making movement even more difficult. Contractures cause a decrease in capillary blood flow to body areas. Research demonstrates a large number of pressure ulcers are the result of some type of contractures.

- Decreased circulation from prolonged immobility magnifies the risk for skin breakdown.

- The lack of activity decreases appetite and slows peristalsis. Clients are at a higher risk for indigestion, heartburn, constipation, and choking.

- The psychological impact of immobility erodes a person's self-esteem. Feelings of helplessness, depression, loneliness, and boredom arise from being inactive.

PRESSURE ULCERS

Lecture Material for Slide 6-4

A pressure ulcer is any lesion caused by unrelieved pressure resulting in damage to underlying tissue. A pressure ulcer is also known as decubitus ulcer, pressure sore, ischemic ulcer, or bedsore. Any compromised body system affects skin integrity. Without proper nutrients, the cells do not have the essential elements to regenerate. Every cell needs water, nutrients, and oxygen to survive.

- Dementia clients are more likely to be sedentary, causing skin breakdown. Pressure ulcers begin as a reddened area, usually over a bony prominence. Without relief from the pressure, the skin continues to be deprived of oxygen and ultimately dies.

- The elderly's skin is thin, cellophanelike, and easily torn or sheared. Health care workers need to be especially careful with aged skin, especially when bathing, dressing, transporting, and pulling clients up in bed. Use a draw sheet to pull the client up in bed to eliminate skin shearing.

- The areas most likely to develop skin breakdown leading to pressure ulcers are the toes, heels, ankles, hips, knees, buttocks, back, shoulders, elbows, and ears. If a reddened area is observed, document the site and notify the supervisor.

- The end-stage dementia client is bed-bound and prone to pressure ulcers. Since the client's immune system is already compromised, the risk of infection is greater. Any signs of infection need to be reported to the supervisor.

- Pad the areas of the client's body where the bones commonly rub together (knees and ankles).
- Bed-bound clients need to be turned at least every two hours. Remind or prompt clients who are chair-bound to reposition themselves every 20 minutes.
- The skin needs to be kept clean and dry. Change the incontinent client when soiled.
- Use facility-approved skin lotion on dry skin areas.
- Keep bed linens clean, as well as free of wrinkles and creases.
- Observe and report any skin changes.
- Check the folds of the skin for breakdown (under breasts, the abdomen, and the groin).

Insert agency's policy for pressure ulcer prevention here.

DEHYDRATION

Dehydration, a condition resulting from the excessive loss of body fluid, may result from fluid deprivation, the excessive loss of fluid, or a reduction in the total quantity of electrolytes.

- The average person consumes approximately two to three liters of fluid daily. The fluid comes from liquid beverages, fruits, and vegetables.
- A common cause of dehydration is vomiting, diarrhea, excessive urination, and body fluid drainage. A person expelling large amounts of electrolytes (sodium and potassium) becomes dehydrated if the electrolytes are not replaced.
- Older adults have a decreased thirst sensation. Others may refuse to drink in order to reduce the incidence of incontinence. Some elderly do not prefer water but are willing to drink other fluids for their daily intake. The dementia client frequently cannot discern the feeling of thirst. Ideational apraxia makes drinking fluids difficult.

Signs of Dehydration

Notify the supervisor if the following signs are noted:

- Dry mucus membranes
- Decreased tearing or salivation
- Coated tongue
- Flushed dry skin (due to the elevated body temperature)
- Concentrated urine or decreased urine output
- Poor skin turgor (elasticity)
- Irritability, confusion, and lethargy (due to fluid and electrolyte imbalances)

Lecture Material for Slide 6-7

INFECTIONS

Infectious disease accounts for a large number of deaths in people 65 years or older. Clients in long-term care facilities and those with underlying health conditions are prone to developing infections.

- The aging client's immune system is compromised due to poor nutrition, dehydration, decreased ambulation, poor oral care, and medication therapy.
- The older adult is at greater risk of developing infections such as pneumonia, influenza, and urinary tract infections.
- The seriousness and acceleration of infections in the elderly may be due to a compromised immune system, drug intolerance, drug toxicity, or multidrug-resistant organisms.
- A systemic infection refers to an infection affecting the whole body.
- An infection can be localized, affecting only one particular tissue or organ.
- A wound infection is the contamination of the broken skin or mucous membranes with an infectious agent.
- Sepsis is an infection that has entered the bloodstream and is life threatening if left untreated.
- The detection of symptoms is frequently masked in the older adult and requires stringent observation. Report any signs and symptoms of an infection to the supervisor.

Signs and Symptoms of Systemic and Wound Infections

- Fever
- Chills
- Redness, pain, and swelling at the wound site
- Heat or warmth at the site
- Purulent or foul smelling drainage at wound site
- Altered mental status and lethargy
- Tachycardia

Lecture Material for Slide 6-8

MEDICATION

Drug therapy in the elderly is complicated by many factors unique to the age group. Many elderly are frail and suffer from multiple medical problems.

- The average older person takes five prescription medications and three over-the-counter drugs. The average institutionalized elderly person is on seven daily medications. Older adults utilize 25% of all prescribed medications. Studies suggest the greater the number of medications used by the elderly population, the higher the incidence of adverse drug reactions.
- Advancing age produces changes in pharmacokinetics (the rate of absorption, distribution, metabolism, and elimination of medication

in the body). These changes increase the susceptibility of adverse drug reactions.

- Drug companies are required to include separate labeling for geriatric clients to ensure the safe and effective use of prescription drugs.

- A large percentage of elderly clients receive inappropriate medications.

- Elderly persons are admitted to hospitals for adverse drug reactions at three times the rate of younger individuals.

- Medications used to treat Alzheimer's disease, comorbid conditions, and behavioral symptoms increase the client's susceptibility to drug reactions.

- In the event of behavioral changes, first consider a medication reaction as the cause. Medications have greatly improved the quality of life for many individuals. The use of drug therapy over time impacts all body systems, some negatively. The benefits of the drugs should surpass their risks. Depending on the client's symptoms, pharmaceutical intervention should be based on individual needs. Monitor the client for medication side-effects and possible drug reactions.

- The caregiver needs to monitor how the side-effects of medications impact all aspects of the client's condition. Observations should include the clients' physical condition, their interactions with others, and their safety in the environment. Interventions may need to be updated to support the client. Report all findings to the supervisor.

Lecture Material for Slide 6-9

● PAIN MANAGEMENT

The feeling of pain, whether abrupt or persistent, can greatly affect the quality of life for individuals. The definition of pain is simply whatever the client says.

- No objective measurement or tests for pain exists; consequently pain is frequently omitted from assessments or treatment plans.

- Some physicians lack adequate knowledge about pain management for the terminally ill. In one study, more than 60% of families felt the individual with dementia was in pain "often" or "all of the time" during the last year of life.

- The interpretation and meaning of pain are very individualized and involve various psychosocial and cultural factors. Clients with dementia may be unable to interpret or communicate their pain or both.

Perception of Pain

- The perception of pain is largely influenced by the cerebral cortex, particularly the parietal lobe. As a result, the pain is the product of a person's past experience, values, cultural expectations, emotions, and the pain stimulus itself.

- With Alzheimer's disease, the area that interprets pain sensation, pressure, temperature, and touch becomes damaged and may greatly affect the client's reaction to pain.

Incidence of Pain

- The incidence of pain is described by the extent or rate of the occurrence.
- Acute pain is relatively short-lived, intense, and reversible. Acute pain alerts the body to an illness or injury. The symptoms of pain are clues to help make a diagnosis.
- Chronic pain serves no useful purpose; it is continuous or habitual. The pain may begin as an acute episode but does not diminish. Another type of chronic pain begins insidiously and slowly over time with increasing intensity. Chronic pain is usually pain persisting longer than six months.

Communication of Pain

- As the disease progresses, AD clients lose the ability to engage in conversation. The behaviors of people with AD say more about what they are feeling than they can express in words. Since they may be unable to communicate, observing for signs of pain may be the only tool available for pain assessment.
- Nonverbal communication can display a person's feelings, comfort, and anxiety. The caregiver should observe the client for any indication of pain.
- Nonverbal communication includes everything that does not involve the spoken or written word: body language (posture and position), tones of voice, gestures, facial expressions, touch, and eye contact.

Signs of Pain

- The most reliable indicator of pain is what is reported by an individual. The effects of AD limit the client's ability to convey pain. The caregiver needs to closely observe for any signs of pain and report it to the supervisor.
- Understanding the client's day-to-day activities, including sleep patterns, relationships with others, and present level of physical activity can contribute to the pain assessment. When certain stressful activities exacerbate the pain, the careplan should be modified.

Audience Interaction for Slide 6-9

Ask the audience to describe the signs of pain commonly exhibited by individuals. Include the following signs of pain in the discussion.

- Increased heart rate, respiratory rate, and blood pressure
- Moans and sighs
- Crying
- Grimacing
- Changes in ambulation or movement
- Rigid posturing
- Withdrawing of extremity when touched
- Changes in muscle tension
- Excessive sweating (diaphoresis).

- Pallor
- Weakness or exhaustion
- Any new behavioral changes

PAIN ASSESSMENT

The key to assessing pain is to pay attention to the client's complaints. Evaluating the pain from the client's perspective enables the caregiver to gain a more accurate assessment. Incorporate daily pain assessment in the plan of care. Assessing pain is considered the fifth vital sign. Gather all data about the pain to assure a viable treatment plan. Inadequate assessment is the principal barrier to pain management.

Observation of Pain

Observation is important when assessing the pain of dementia clients. When communication skills are limited, the physical signs of pain need to validate the complaints.

- Try to determine the location of the pain. Superficial pain is easier to locate. Have the client point to the site or place the client's hand on the suspected area.
- Based on observations or the client's description, determine the type of pain. Types of pain may be described as localized, diffuse, referred, or radiating.
- The quality of pain is another subjective characteristic. A client may describe the pain as crushing, throbbing, sharp, dull, or burning.
- Have the client rate the pain on a scale from one to five (five being the worst) or another descriptive scale that the client can understand. Pictures may be useful. The FlACC Pain Scale may be helpful for the dementia client since the observed categories use nonverbal behaviors. Determine what works best for the client and communicate to everyone involved with care. Increasing pain may be a sign of a worsening condition.
- Determine whether the pain is acute or chronic and when it began. Acute pain may be the outcome of an infection, while the chronic pain of osteoarthritis, for example, calls for a different treatment plan.
- Determine how pain affects the client's everyday routine. Does he or she stop participating in social events? Is there a change in eating patterns? Is the client experiencing new behaviors or challenges?
- Observe what triggers the client's pain. Does the client complain of leg pain after going for a walk? Does the client become restless before going to the bathroom?
- Observe for the effects of any treatment regime prescribed. Monitor the client for adverse reactions to pain medication. The sedative effect can alter the level of consciousness. Safety concerns, such as falls, may need to be addressed.
- Notify the supervisor of any changes in the client's condition.

Lecture Material for Slide 6-12

TREATMENTS FOR PAIN

Pain is a preventable health issue, which diminishes a person's quality of life. Eliminating pain should be part of the entire care planning process. The overall goal of pain management is to decrease and ultimately eliminate pain.

Pharmacological Treatments

- The use of pharmacological treatments is an accepted form of pain management.

- When medications are prescribed for pain management, they should be administered as directed. By keeping to the schedule, a steady blood level of medication is maintained, limiting the "peaks and valleys" of pain control.

- Chronic pain requires around-the-clock medication minimizing side-effects and producing a steady stream of medicine. The client does not have the pain because the pain medication is working. Administer medication before the pain returns.

- Breakthrough pain should be treated as needed. Increasing pain is a sign that the disease is worsening.

- When clients are independent in administering medications, remind them of the time schedule and the side-effects.

- Clients and families may be hesitant to request pain medication for fear of addiction. Studies have shown that very few people become addicted to the medications when treating a terminal illness. Studies also suggest hospitalized Alzheimer's clients are less medicated and suffer from pain more than when residing at home.

- Monitor the client for adverse reactions to all medications.

Comfort Measures

Sufferers of chronic pain may benefit from the addition of nonpharmacological approaches and comfort measures. Comfort measures are interventions aimed at reducing pain and relieving symptoms. Methods may be traditional or holistic in nature. Client comfort is a significant health care goal.

- The use of comfort measures is a common and approved practice. The rationale for the use of comfort measures is to decrease pain, anxiety, and fear for the client.

- A touch, a rub, or the sound of soft music are methods used to reduce client's anxiety, thereby aiding in minimizing pain.

- Many times comfort measures are used as a distraction.

- Optimally, attempt to use pre-illness preferences and incorporate with the comfort measures.

Examples of commonly used comfort approaches are:

- Back rubs.
- Reading to the client.
- Listening to music.

- Bringing in a favorite blanket.
- Breathing exercises.
- Aromatherapy.

Audience Interaction for Slide 6-12

Ask the audience for additional helpful strategies in reducing pain.

Lecture Material for Slides 6-13 and 6-14

● REVIEW OF END-STAGE ALZHEIMER'S DISEASE

In the late stage of dementia, the brain no longer has the capacity to tell the mind to think, the soul to feel, or the body to move. According to the staging protocol of the Global Deterioration Scale (GDS) developed by Dr. Barry Reisberg, severe dementia is known as stage seven.

Slide 6-13

Symptoms of Late-Stage AD

- Cognitive dysfunction is very severe (clients need all ADL performed for them).
- Communication is limited to grunting.
- Basic psychomotor skills are lost (the client is unable to walk, sit up without assistance, and has little head control).
- Clients seek immediate sensory gratification and can easily be overstimulated.
- Clients are very resistant to unfamiliar persons providing personal care.
- Resistant to unfamiliar persons.

Slide 6-14

- Clients accept some interaction but will not initiate them.
- The eyes are no longer able to focus.
- Infant reflexes such as rooting, sucking, grasping, and the Babinski sign return (the brain deterioration causes the body to return to the infancy state).
- The brain stem is invaded with plaques and tangles. (The brain stem controls the involuntary functions of breathing, blinking, blood pressure, and other vital body functions. Without the functions of the brain stem, the body dies without extraordinary means).
- Brain stem involvement.

Lecture Material for Slide 6-15

● END-OF-LIFE (EOL) CARE AND DEMENTIA

Dying is part of life, which brings about contemplation of personal issues and beliefs. Also, this reminds everyone of his or her own mortality. End-of-life (EOL) care is the care of an individual during the last phase of life. Alzheimer's disease, in its advanced stage, becomes a terminal illness.

During the late stage of the disease the client is unable to recognize loved ones, communicate, ambulate, and control bowel or bladder functions. When the client begins to lose weight and has difficulties swallowing, the prognosis of death is within two years regardless of medical interventions.

- Once family members can accept the advanced stage of Alzheimer's as terminal, palliative care or supportive measures can be instituted.
- In a study on death and dying of AD clients, more than 90% of the caregivers felt death came as a relief to the AD victim. Seventy-two percent felt it was a relief to them.
- Death is a subject of much controversy; religious leaders, philosophers, and political ideologies all ponder its meaning.
- The perceptions of death and expressions of grief vary by age, culture, past experience, support systems, and spiritual beliefs. Spiritual beliefs include practices, rites, and rituals directed toward the loss and grieving process.
- Behaviors of grief may not indicate the true feelings of the bereaved but rather the expectation of the person's culture.

General Components of EOL Care

End-of-life care differs from traditional care by including the client, family, and caregiver. The AD client is spared the end-of-life social isolation, psychological stress, and spiritual crisis.

Symptom Management

- Symptom control is an essential component of quality EOL care. Pain is a real phenomenon to a dying client.
- Clients experience many of the same symptoms regardless of the underlying disease process. The symptoms add to their suffering and their families' suffering.
- Report all observations to the supervisor.

Common EOL Symptoms

- Pain
- Difficulty breathing (dyspnea)
- Confusion
- Loss of appetite and muscle wasting (cachexia)
- Nausea
- Fatigue
- Depression

Goals of EOL Care

- The goals of care are specific treatment choices encountered during the end of life.
- Advanced planning is essential for fulfilling end-of-life wishes. The physicians and health care team should initiate discussions with the

- individual and family regarding their wishes. Early discussion helps to clarify the individual's requests before the onset of severe dementia.
- The pattern of decline for the AD client differs dramatically among individuals depending on where the tangles develop. The only constant is that the AD client dies. Families and caregivers need to be proactive, making decisions when the client is lucid and competent.
- Whether to use do not resuscitate (DNR) orders or life-sustaining treatments (tube feeding or ventilators) must be determined as part of the treatment plan.

Palliative Care

- Palliative care is the use of therapies designed to relieve or reduce the intensity of symptoms but is not curative.
- Palliative care is not the same as extraordinary measures or experimental treatments. The essence of palliative care is to allow the client to be more comfortable and have a better quality of the end of their life.
- Palliative treatments include any treatments, medical equipment, tests, procedures, and medication necessary to provide high-quality comfort care.

Hospice

- Hospice is a form of palliative care that uses a multidisciplinary team approach (doctors, nurses, HCA, volunteers, social workers, chaplains, and bereavement counselors) when treating the dying client. The mission of hospice is to allow everyone the right to die pain free and with dignity. The focus is on caring, not curing. Hospice services require the client's prognosis to be less than six months.
- The elements of hospice include maintaining comfort through all means of pain relief and symptom control. Bereavement support for the family continues after the death of the client.
- Most of hospice care is provided in the client's home. Hospice care also takes place in freestanding hospice facilities, hospitals, and long-term care facilities.
- Most health insurance and Medicare cover hospice services.

Communication

- Communication is an important component of EOL care. No matter what the goals of care or the disease process, open communication is essential.
- With Alzheimer's disease, the client's ability to communicate lessens. Continue to speak to and explain treatments even when the client becomes unresponsive.
- The remaining focus should be centered on the family's needs to accept the outcome.
- Caring for the client with AD becomes a large part of the families' life. The "long death" may cause caregivers to grieve with every functional loss. End-of-life care impacts formal and informal caregivers.

Audience Interaction for Slide 6-15

- Arrange for families and caregivers to discuss their fears and concerns. Encourage the expression of feelings by listening.

Ask the audience to explore their personal feelings about death. Include the following in the discussion:

- The right things to say or do are not always known.
- Treat the client as "you" would want to be treated.
- Show compassion for the client and family.
- Be confident in the care provided.
- Listen to the family and client's concerns. Offering care and support to a family during the end of life can be very rewarding.

Lecture Material for Slide 6-16

IMPENDING DEATH

When death is near, physical changes occur to prepare the body to cease functioning. Not all symptoms are experienced by every dying client, and no specific order of symptoms exists. The caregiver should provide comfort measures to the client and the family. Maintain a neat and clean room. Air the room of any odors; change bed linens when soiled. Most importantly respect the client's and family's privacy and wishes.

Signs and Symptoms of Impending Death

- The extremities become cool and may have a bluish hue.
- Clients may experience chills and sweating.
- The client sleeps most of the time and may become unresponsive.
- The normal cognitive disturbance associated with death is not apparent in the dementia client. Any communication skills or verbalization lessen.
- Pain is apparently absent.
- Any remaining bladder or bowel control ceases.
- The client has an increase in congestion or makes gurgling noises, commonly referred to as the death rattle.
- The client becomes increasingly restless.
- Urinary output decreases.
- Appetite and thirst are absent.
- When the end is near, the client's breathing patterns change to shallow breaths with periods of apnea or no breaths (Cheyne-Stokes breathing).

Interventions to Support the Dying Client

- The client should be kept clean, warm, and dry. Change any damp or soiled clothing or linens. Personal care should be maintained.
- Use protective items to keep linens from being soiled.

- To avoid skin breakdown, reposition the client as tolerated. Use pillows or other mechanical devices to provide comfort.
- Explain all interventions to the client even though there is no response.
- Notify the supervisor of any alteration in the client's respiratory status, including congestion.
- Turn the client's head to the side to allow secretions to drain. Wipe the draining secretions from the mouth.
- Monitor the client's urinary output.
- Do not force food or fluids. Reassure the family that the client no longer feels hunger or needs nutrients.
- Provide comfort measures for dry mouth and lips (eg, ice chips, glycerin swabs).
- Use tranquil music, light massage, a soothing voice to reduce the restlessness.

Death of the Client

Insert agency's policy regarding pronouncements here.

Signs of Death

- Breathing stops.
- The heartbeat stops.
- The client cannot be aroused.
- The eyelids may be partially or fully open, and the eyes are fixed.
- The mouth may be slightly open.
- The release of urine and stool.

Preparing the Body after Death

Insert agency's policy regarding postmortem care here.

SUMMING UP

Through the progression of Alzheimer's disease, emerging medical conditions may impact the quality of life and contribute to the death of the individual. Since Alzheimer's disease occurs in the latter half of life, the changes impact all body systems and functions. Aging and illness can affect the presentation of symptoms, the response to treatment, and outcomes.

The AD client is more prone to certain medical conditions due to the insidiousness of the disease. Conditions such as dehydration, injuries, infection, pneumonia, constipation, and complications associated with immobility have a serious impact on the dementia client. When developing treatment plans, the stage of dementia and the medical conditions should both be considered.

The assessment and treatment of pain are difficult for the caregiver, and special interventions need to be included in the plan of care for the cognitively impaired client. Decreasing pain increases a client's quality of life.

End-of-life care is as important to the family and client as life care. Treat the client and family as "you" would like to be treated. The end of life means different things to different people. Everyone should talk to loved ones about end-of-life decisions and wishes. Discuss any concerns with the supervisor regarding the caregiver's role and EOL care. Most important, enjoy each day and live life.

Instructor's Version with Answers for Handout 6-4

● REAL-LIFE SCENARIO

A Day in the Life of Pat

Pat is in the latter stage of AD and has poor mobility. Pat is confined to a wheelchair. According to the staff, Pat has a decreased appetite and refuses to drink when the health care team offers liquids. Pat enjoys limited foods and is eating less at meals.

1. What medical problems is Pat predisposed to given the information?
   - *Constipation*
   - *Pressure ulcers*
   - *Dehydration*
   - *Infections leading to pneumonia*

2. What signs of body system changes should Pat's caregiver observe?

   The caregiver should observe the client for the following signs of body system changes:
   - *Changes in behavior.*
   - *Increased agitation.*
   - *Nausea or vomiting.*
   - *Diarrhea.*
   - *Skin changes.*
   - *Coughing.*
   - *Respiratory congestion.*
   - *Increased lethargy.*
   - *Changes in gait.*
   - *Swelling of any extremity.*

3. What are the complications from immobility?

   Complications of immobility include:
   - *An increased risk of pulmonary complications.*
   - *An increased threat of a thrombus or an embolus.*
   - *Edema of the dependent extremities.*
   - *Muscle weakness and atrophy.*
   - *Muscle contractors or deformities.*
   - *Skin breakdown and pressure ulcers.*
   - *Indigestion, heartburn, constipation, and choking.*
   - *Feelings of helplessness, depression, loneliness, and boredom.*

GROUP ACTIVITY

● PURPOSE OF THE ACTIVITY

The purpose of this activity is to explore possible ways of identifying pain in the client with dementia. The following activities can be completed as a class, in small groups, or individually.

Each participant role-plays as a caregiver and as a client with dementia. Have the student dementia client choose an acute and chronic pain, imitating the deficits commonly seen with a dementia client. Through observation, have the student caregiver determine the location, type, and cause of the pain. Reverse the roles and repeat.

Name _____ Date _____

Program/Course _____ Instructor's Name _____

Common Medical Problems Pre- and Post-Test

1. The process of normal aging, in the absence of disease, is accompanied by vast changes affecting all body systems. What change is not part of the normal aging process?
   a. Appearance
   b. Intelligence
   c. Vision
   d. Hormone levels

2. During the course of AD, clients may develop additional medical conditions. Name three common conditions.
   a. Dehydration, vitreous floaters, and acne
   b. Dyspnea, hypothyroidism, and osteoporosis
   c. Dehydration, constipation, and pressure ulcers
   d. Dyspnea, constipation, and pressure ulcers

3. When assessing a dementia client for pain, the caregiver should:
   a. Frequently ask the client if he or she is experiencing pain.
   b. Observe the client's nonverbal communication for signs of pain.
   c. Omit a pain assessment since the dementia client no longer has pain.
   d. Distract the client.

4. Define end-of-life care.
   a. The care of the body after the person has died
   b. The care given to a person during the dying process
   c. The spiritual needs provided at the time of the person's death
   d. The signs and symptoms of approaching death

5. What are the symptoms of late-stage Alzheimer's disease?
   a. Moderately severe cognitive decline, inability to name relevant aspects of their lives, need for some assistance for survival
   b. Mild cognitive decline, manifest deficits in more than one area, and the start of decline in work-related performance
   c. Severe cognitive decline, no orientation to time and place, and incontinence
   d. Very severe cognitive decline, little or no communication, no basic psychomotor skills, the presence of infant reflexes

Handout **6-1**

THE AGING PROCESS

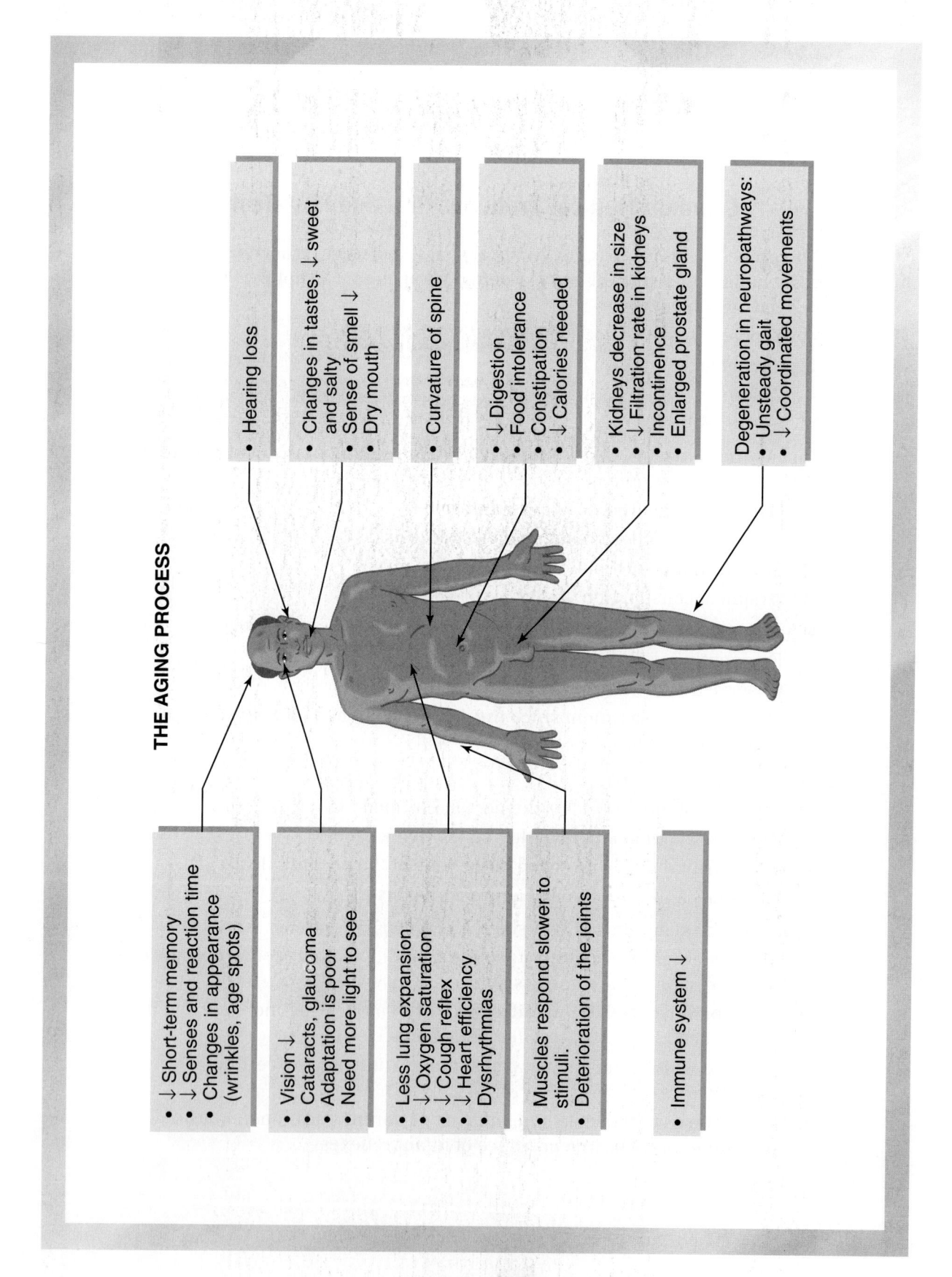

- Hearing loss

- Changes in tastes, ↓ sweet and salty
- Sense of smell ↓
- Dry mouth

- Curvature of spine

- ↓ Digestion
- Food intolerance
- Constipation
- ↓ Calories needed

- Kidneys decrease in size
- ↓ Filtration rate in kidneys
- Incontinence
- Enlarged prostate gland

- Degeneration in neuropathways:
- Unsteady gait
- ↓ Coordinated movements

- ↓ Short-term memory
- ↓ Senses and reaction time
- Changes in appearance (wrinkles, age spots)

- Vision ↓
- Cataracts, glaucoma
- Adaptation is poor
- Need more light to see

- Less lung expansion
- ↓ Oxygen saturation
- ↓ Cough reflex
- ↓ Heart efficiency
- Dysrhythmias

- Muscles respond slower to stimuli.
- Deterioration of the joints

- Immune system ↓

Handout **6-2**

Normal Aging Versus Dementia

Action	Normal Aging	Dementia
ADL	Independent	Dependent
Memory loss	Yes Remembers details of event	Yes Has no memory of event
Friends/family concerned with memory loss	No	Yes
Forgets recent events	No	Yes
Communication skills	No deficits	Deficits noted
Interpersonal skills	Maintained	Limits interactions
Gets lost in familiar areas	No	Yes
Uses appliances	No difficulties	Unable to use
Cognitive function evaluation	Within normal limits	Below normal limits

Handout **6-3**

A Day in the Life of Pat: A Real-Life Scenario

Pat is in the latter stage of AD and has poor mobility. Pat is confined to a wheelchair. According to the staff, Pat has a decreased appetite and refuses to drink when the health care team offers liquids. Pat enjoys limited foods and is eating less at meals.

1. What medical problems is Pat predisposed to, given the information?

2. What signs of body system changes should Pat's caregiver observe?

3. What are the complications from immobility?

Handout **6-4**

MODULE 6 COMMON MEDICAL PROBLEMS

The Normal Aging Process

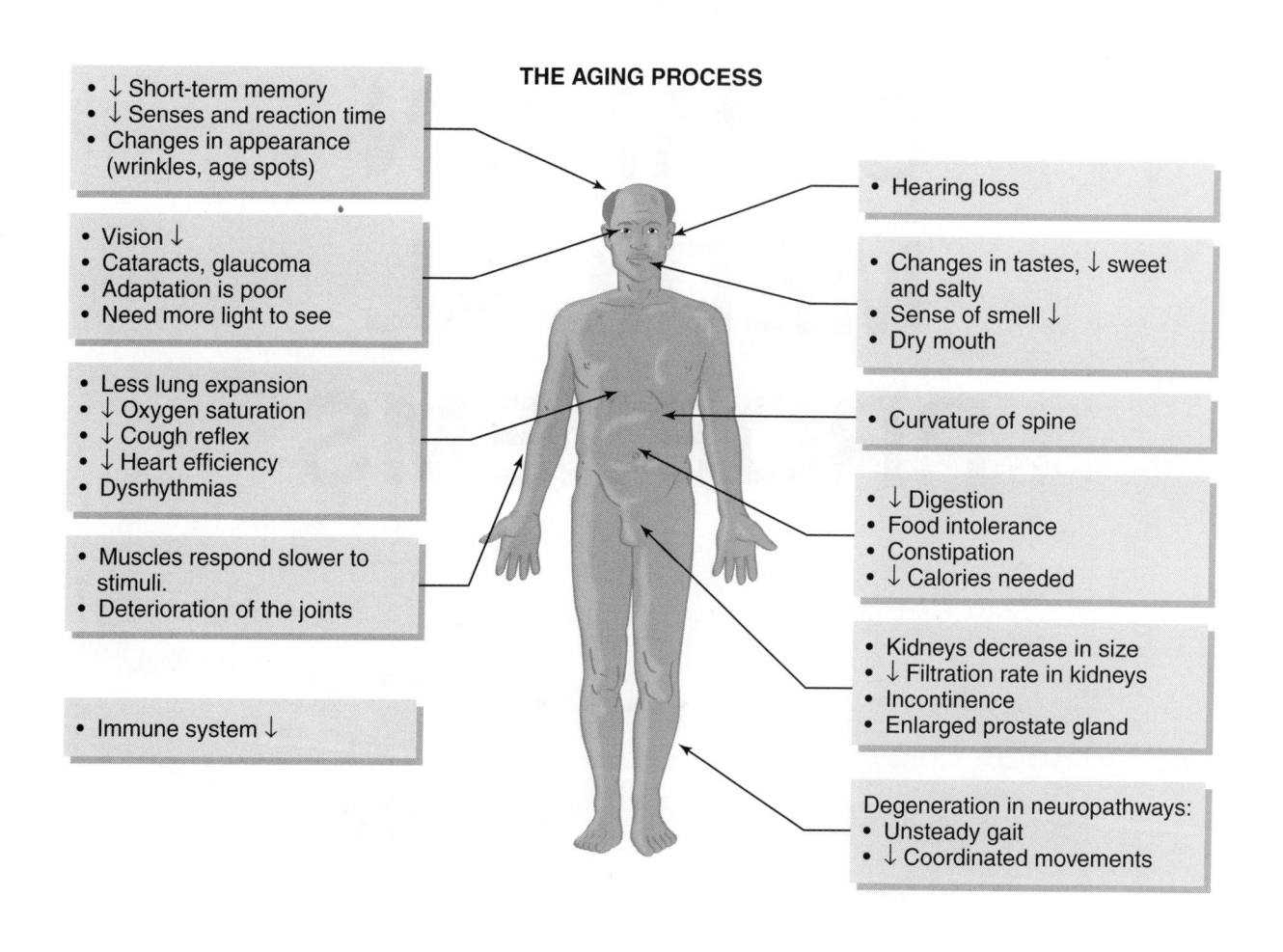

THE AGING PROCESS

- ↓ Short-term memory
- ↓ Senses and reaction time
- Changes in appearance (wrinkles, age spots)

- Vision ↓
- Cataracts, glaucoma
- Adaptation is poor
- Need more light to see

- Less lung expansion
- ↓ Oxygen saturation
- ↓ Cough reflex
- ↓ Heart efficiency
- Dysrhythmias

- Muscles respond slower to stimuli.
- Deterioration of the joints

- Immune system ↓

- Hearing loss

- Changes in tastes, ↓ sweet and salty
- Sense of smell ↓
- Dry mouth

- Curvature of spine

- ↓ Digestion
- Food intolerance
- Constipation
- ↓ Calories needed

- Kidneys decrease in size
- ↓ Filtration rate in kidneys
- Incontinence
- Enlarged prostate gland

- Degeneration in neuropathways:
- Unsteady gait
- ↓ Coordinated movements

Common Medical Problems

- **Dehydration**
- **Unreported injuries**
- **Infections**
- **Pneumonia**
- **Constipation**
- **Complications from prolonged immobility**

Potential Areas for Pressure Ulcers

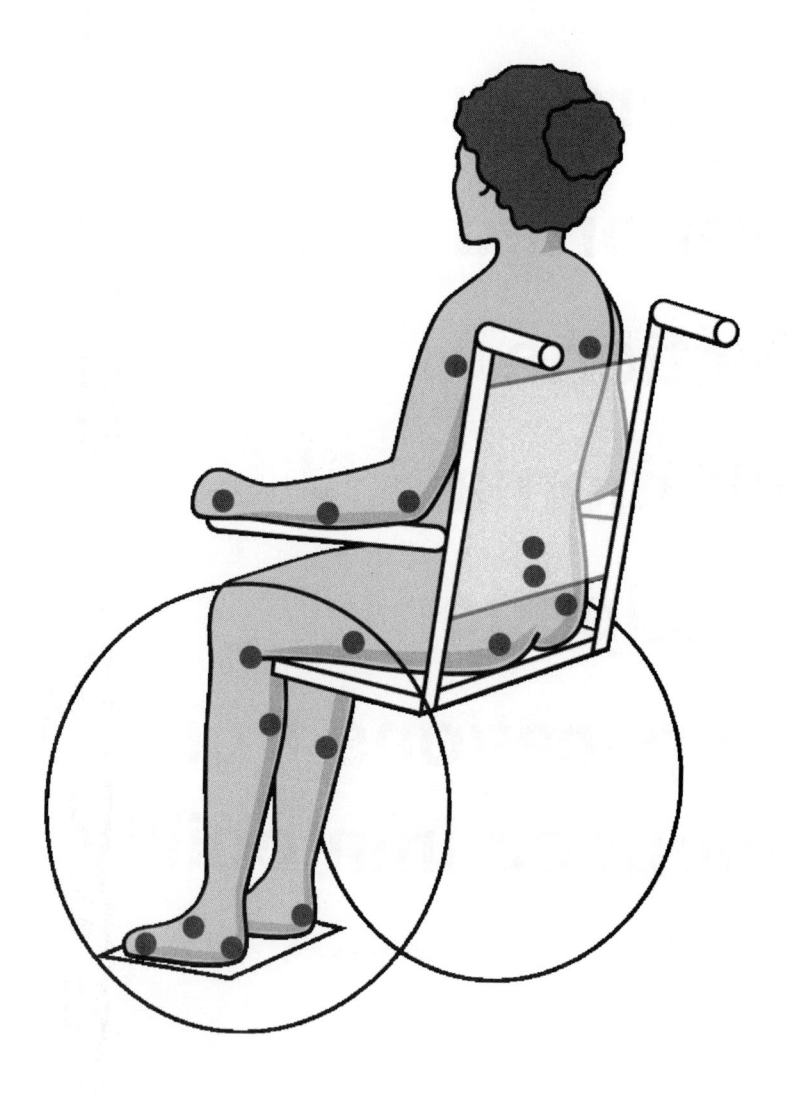

Signs of Dehydration

- **Dry mucus membranes**
- **Decreased tearing or salivation**
- **Coated tongue**
- **Flushed dry skin**

Signs of Dehydration (*cont.*)

- Concentrated urine or decreased urine output
- Poor skin turgor
- Irritability, confusion and lethargy

Signs and Symptoms of Infection

- Fever and chills
- Redness, pain, heat, swelling at site
- Purulent drainage at site
- Altered mental status
- Tachycardia

Medications

Observe and report:
- side effects
- possible drug reactions
- behavioral changes

Pain Management

- **Perception**
- **Incidence**
- **Communication**
- **Signs**

Pain Assessment
The 5th Vital Sign

Observe for:
- **location of pain**
- **type of pain**
- **quality of pain**
- **rating of pain (pain scale)**

Pain Assessment (cont.)

- acute or chronic pain
- effects of pain on ADL
- triggers for pain
- outcomes of treatment regimes

Treatments for Pain

- **Pharmacological**
  - remind clients to take medications
  - monitor side effects
- **Comfort measures**

Symptoms of Late Stage AD

- **Very severe cognitive dysfunction**
- **Little or no communication**
- **No basic psychomotor skills**
- **Seeks immediate gratification**
- **Resistant to unfamiliar persons**

Symptoms of Late Stage AD (cont.)

- **Unable to initiate interaction**
- **Unable to focus**
- **Return of infant reflexes**
- **Brain stem involvement**

Components of EOL Care

- **Symptom management**
- **Goals of care**
- **Communication**

Interventions to Support the Dying Client

- **Keep client clean and dry**
- **Explain all procedures**
- **Monitor respiratory status and urinary output**
- **Do not force food or fluids**
- **Provide comfort measures**

Module 7
Coping with Dementia

Goal
To educate the students how a client copes with dementia.

Objectives
After completion of the presentation, students will be able to:
- Describe how the diagnosis of Alzheimer's disease impacts the client, family, and society.
- List common emotions experienced by the dementia client.
- Describe how the diagnosis of Alzheimer's disease impacts the client and family's role.
- Explain the stages of grief.
- Define a durable power of attorney.
- Describe care options for clients and their families.

GENERAL INFORMATION AND OVERVIEW

Lecture Material for Slide 7-1

As the population ages, the incidence of Alzheimer's disease becomes greater. The average life span following the diagnosis of AD is eight to 10 years, during which time the client suffers a loss of mental faculties related to memory, personality, and behavior. Currently, in the United States 4.5 million people have a diagnosis of AD and the yearly monetary cost of AD exceeds $100 billion. The social and emotional toll is immeasurable, affecting more than just individuals, families, and caregivers but society as well. (NIA)

- The symptoms of Alzheimer's disease initially are perceived more as a nuisance than a concern. Many times the family is unaware of the mild impairment. The client often covers up the memory loss.
- The signs and symptoms of AD begin slowly. The person may forget a familiar place, a person's name, or recent events. The act of forgetting a single incident is not a sign of dementia.
- As the disease progresses, all higher brain functions diminish. Any task requiring executive functioning (the ability to follow a series of steps) and/or abstract thinking (the ability to think in terms of ideas) amplifies the defect. For example, a person has difficulty setting the table for a meal, planning a vacation, or interacting with others.
- Family and friends frequently avoid the term "Alzheimer's disease" when in the client's company. Discussing the AD diagnosis permits clients and families to plan health care decisions. The knowledge of the AD diagnosis may eliminate the client's need to conceal the memory loss.
- An important role in treating AD is early diagnosis. Care options and treatment decisions should be discussed early on in the disease, when the client's decision-making skills are still intact.

Audience Interaction for Slide 7-1

Ask the audience for ways in which Alzheimer's disease affects individuals, families, caregivers, and society. Include the following in the discussion:

- Medical cost.
- Missed work and productivity.
- Loss of interaction with friends.
- Unexpected changes in a preexisting role and social activities.
- Physical demands for caregivers, who are on-call 24 hours a day.
- The need for caregivers to learn basic nursing skills.
- The emotional issues related to caring for someone with a terminal illness.
- Financial impact.

EARLY IN THE DISEASE PROCESS

Lecture Material for Slides 7-2 and 7-3

Slide 7-2

Neuron death begins slowly and continues for many years before any dementia symptoms are noticed. The human brain has the ability to compensate for brain cell death. Research has shown a deterioration of function will appear only after 30% of brain cell loss occurs. Cognitive function changes affect more than just intellect. Client's emotions and relationships are affected. The critical component of dementia is the severe enough loss of intellect to interfere with social and occupational abilities.

Ask the audience to explore possible emotions felt by an individual who just received a diagnosis of AD. Keep track of the answers for a later discussion.

Audience Interaction for Slides 7-2 and 7-3

Trivializing the Memory Loss

- Early in the disease process clients blame others or trivialize the memory loss. Friends and family are able to notice the cognitive changes.
- Initially, the early signs are mistaken for stress and depression. Clients have described the beginning stages by saying, "I knew something was wrong, thoughts would just leave my mind and I was unable to get them back." "I am involved with so many things, and no one in my position could keep everything straight."
- Some may conceal the signs or cover up their forgetfulness. The professor can no longer teach from memory; he needs to write notes to recall the lecture material.

Unaware of the Progressing Condition

- Inevitably, all AD clients become unaware of their progressing condition. The businessperson may make reckless investments and lose a life savings. The housewife may be cooking and forget to turn off the stove. The woman may drive to the store and forget her way home. Interventions are needed to prevent potentially harmful events.
- A sense of complacency among clients with early AD is common. Individuals quickly forget any thoughts of loss and are able to carry on without disappointment.

Varying Perception of Symptoms

- Many clients do not grasp the full implications of the disease, possibly the only saving grace of the illness. Some are relieved by the diagnosis and less embarrassed by their behavior and need for help.
- The awareness of memory loss varies greatly; some have insight into their disability while others do not. A majority of affected individuals have fluctuations in their awareness. They become aware only when faced with a task that is far beyond their abilities.
- Clients who are oblivious to their symptoms are not in denial. Memory and judgment difficulties result in their forgetting about forgetting. Orienting or confronting people about their limitations or failures does not improve their symptoms but frequently becomes upsetting for all involved. One client states, "You cannot experience what you have forgotten."
- For those who are unaware of their symptoms, any initiation of assistance may be regarded as unnecessary, demeaning, and intrusive.

- The true nature of the disease often diminishes the awareness of the severity of symptoms and reduces the person's ability to see issues clearly.
- Symptom awareness may be related to the amount of damage to the frontal lobe, which controls awareness and judgment.

Concerns about Making Mistakes

- When clients have insight into their limitations they accept help as necessary. The knowledge of symptoms causes them to feel self-conscious and worry about making mistakes in public. For the minority of those who are aware of their symptoms, every day can be a frustrating series of failures.
- Some clients with AD feel conflicted about asking or receiving help. One person writes, "I feel I am not my own person anymore."
- Frequently, clients with early-stage AD have limited insight into how the disease affects their lives. Most people do not dwell on their impairments or find ways to excuse them.

Slide 7-3

Suspicion, Loneliness, and Fear

- Many clients affected with dementia express feelings of loneliness and alienation. Clients state they feel alone in the world, "No one really knows what's going on." Additional statements include: "I miss being important," "I miss being needed," or "I am so alone and we don't know what's going on in ourselves."
- Fear is a predominant complaint of clients, a sense of dread never experienced before.
- Persons become irrational due to fear or feeling left out. One woman stated she constantly needs assurance from her husband that he will not leave her.
- Suspicion and paranoia are commonly observed with the dementia client.

Impact on Social Activities

- The loss of communication skills impacts social companionship and interactions. Following a diagnosis of AD, many clients experience a loss of friends. "No one wants to talk to you any longer." "It is easier for me to stay home than go out where people don't understand me and judge me . . . maybe it would be easier if I didn't look healthy."
- Because of the disease process, clients are unable to hide their true feelings.
- Feelings of self are threatened when connections with people, places, and things are separated. Studies show the lack of self-awareness and personal identity lead to physical deterioration and a vegetative state. The essence of dementia care is to maintain a connection to the client.

Live in the Here and Now

- Despite the awareness of their symptoms and changing environment, most clients are able to adapt. They begin to look at the world again as though it was for the first time. Clients live in the moment and enjoy the littlest of things as seen through a child's eyes. One client wrote, "I am more patient and take things slower."

- The inability to recall the past or plans for the future allows the dementia client to focus on the present and distant past. Clients no longer have to deliberate on the responsibility of remembering and planning; they just experience the "here and now."

- The quality of life for cognitively impaired clients is improved by understanding the person behind the dementia.

Audience Interaction for Slides 7-2 and 7-3

Refer to the responses offered in the previous audience interaction regarding the possible emotions felt by an individual who just received a diagnosis of AD and compare with the preceding lecture material. Share how answers differ. Include in the discussion how past experiences and memory hinder the insight into how the disease affects clients.

Lecture Material for Slides 7-4 through 7-6

Slide 7-4

● CHANGES IN ROLE

The deterioration and loss of neurons are the basis of the short-term memory loss. The client is unable to take new information and integrate it with facts already learned. When AD clients are no longer equipped to manage their environment or role in society, others need to assume authority, creating a shift in role. Learning new roles is difficult for the individual taking on the new responsibility, as well as for clients having to relinquish their responsibility.

- When a family member becomes ill, the roles in the family change. Roles and responsibilities are different for everyone. A role is the part played in society: mother, father, daughter, teacher, and caregiver. The wife who was the homemaker now is responsible for becoming the breadwinner.

- When the time comes to relinquish responsibilities (balancing a checkbook or driving), the person with AD begins to feel useless, frustrated, and depressed. "I always took care of the family, now I can't do anything." Acknowledging the client's declining health is problematic for the entire family.

- An individual's social role is attained by the extent of their participation in society. Interpersonal skills diminish with AD, decreasing socializing. They withdraw from social events and no longer can participate in conversations.

- Clients are unable to keep up with new developments in their profession and unable to discuss current events. The social bowler may no longer play in the league for fear of not being able to keep score. The grandmother who knits may lose her interest in the craft when she can no longer remember the stitches. A professor is unable to remember lesson plans, student's names, and the repetitive requirements of the job.

- The dementia client may become easily agitated with changes in the environment. The grandmother may wake up confused and anxious when visiting the daughter's home.
- The dementia client begins to have difficulty finding the correct word (anomia). Initially the person tries to hide the word searching difficulty by describing the word. The woman at the restaurant, forgetting the word "knife," asks the waiter for the implement needed to cut her food.
- When others see and notice the forgetfulness and inability to perform common tasks, medical treatment is usually sought. Clients are aware of the changes but fear and anxiety prevent them from seeking medical treatment. A wife, hearing the diagnosis, says, "He was always a happy person, then he became withdrawn and maudlin." The embarrassment and fear of an impending diagnosis at times prevent clients from talking about their suspicions.

The diagnosis of AD is daunting and frightening, and it brings about extreme life changes for friends and families. Clients' cognitive resources and the behavioral approaches used to manage emotional demands are exceeding their abilities. Increasing social support and coping skills minimize stress. The expectations of others must adjust to the client's declining abilities. New tasks must be learned and mastered. One woman states, describing a loved one with AD, "We are the ones who must change. He cannot and will not change to suit us."

Slide 7-5

When the Client Is a Parent

- The diagnosis of AD for a parent changes the parent-child relationship forever. When a child must care for an ill parent, psychologists refer to this as role reversal. The parent was the one who always cared for the child. The child may lack confidence in accepting the parental role. "How can I tell mom she shouldn't drive?"
- Adult children have feelings of loss when a parent is diagnosed with AD. The child has lost a source of support they have relied on for most of his or her life.
- The child must take on additional unpleasant duties, which become burdensome. Role reversal may cause feelings of resentment.

Slide 7-6

Audience Interaction for Slide 7-6

Read the following scenario to the audience and discuss how changes in role impact family dynamics.

A family is preparing for a holiday dinner. Vincent struggles with the holiday decorations and he throws them down in frustration. Loretta begins to sob while watching the man who has shared her life for 40 years slipping away. Her role as a caregiver comes to fruition.

When the Client Is a Spouse

- The affect of AD on a partnership varies depending on the dynamics of the pre-illness relationship. A leadership role must be maintained. The transition of leadership can evolve as the disease progresses.
- When the AD client can no longer manage the role of the provider, head of the household, or homemaker, the partner absorbs the responsibilities. The caregiver needs to take on the other partner's role as well as his or her own.
- Many caregivers become overwhelmed and sad at the reality of the situation. The disease process and loss of companionship add to the burden of the new roles.

Lecture Material for Slide 7-7

RESPONSES TO THE DIAGNOSIS OF DEMENTIA

Grief is the physical and emotional response to loss, death, or separation. When experiencing a loss, grief is a natural reaction. Behaviors and feelings associated with the grieving process occur differently in individuals. The diagnosis of AD brings and creates a multitude of losses for both the client and family. Feelings of sorrow, loneliness, sadness, shame, and guilt emerge in families living with a diagnosis of dementia.

Stages of Grief

Theories of the grieving process are used to assist the health care team in dealing with the emotional needs of the client and family. Many theories have been developed defining the grieving process and reactions to loss. Grieving theories help health care providers understand how loss affects behaviors. Dr. Elisabeth Kubler-Ross, well known for her research on death and dying, believes the process of grief has distinctive phases or stages. Anyone experiencing loss encounters some form of grief. The stages may not be easy to identify for each person and may occur in different orders. Everyone grieves in his or her own way.

Denial and Isolation Stage

In the denial and isolation stage, the individual refuses to believe or understand that a loss has occurred. The belief shields a person against the shock of dying or losing someone. Denial is often a healthy defense mechanism by helping the person cope with the devastating news. The shock and isolation allow the person time to become accustomed to the loss before responding to the reality of the situation.

- Upon being diagnosed, the family of the AD client may not want to believe the diagnosis. "The doctor must be wrong, my husband has just been under a lot of stress." Many times the client and the family cannot comprehend the true impact of the situation. The diagnosis in most cases puts the family onto an emotional roller coaster.

- During this phase clients may become apprehensive about asking for assistance for fear of rejection, therefore isolating themselves from others. One of the barriers about asking for help is that clients may be looking inward and experiencing negative feelings about themselves. Most people find it difficult understanding that asking for help does not indicate weakness or failure.

Anger Stage

In this stage the person resists the loss. The person acts out and becomes angry at the world. Frequent outbursts or ventings of emotion are common. The anger can stem from added demands or from feelings of abandonment.

- Family members are often the recipients of misdirected anger from the dementia client.
- Terror and helplessness are coupled with feelings of injustice and unfairness.
- To find meaning to this fate, some people internalize their feelings and irrationally conclude they have brought the disease on themselves by bad behavior. "This happened to our family because we were never there for other people when they needed our help."
- The anger generated by the situation is enough to push the family into a deep depression. Families are sometimes unable to help the client because of their own anger.

Bargaining Stage

In the bargaining stage the person tries to postpone the reality of the loss. The individual may attempt to "make a deal" to prevent the loss from occurring. Frequently the opinions of others are sought out during this stage.

- The dementia client and their family may call on their deity for help.
- Second and third opinions may be sought in the hope that the diagnosis is incorrect.

Depression Stage

During this stage the person begins to realize the full impact of the loss. Frequently, feelings of depression arise after a significant decline in the client's condition. Overwhelming feelings of loneliness and a withdrawal from social interactions follow. The depression stage provides an opportunity to work through the loss and begin the process of problem solving.

Acceptance Stage

In the final stage of the grieving process, acceptance is reached. The reality of the loss is recognized. The person comes to terms with the situation, no longer feeling hopeless. The acceptance stage occurs only with individuals who have time to work through the other stages of grief.

⬤ EMOTIONS AND DEMENTIA

Lecture Material for Slide 7-8

The diagnosis of AD alters the moods of both the client and those around them. The client and family experience the waxing and waning of emotions during their journey.

Depression

- Depression is commonly witnessed in the wake of a life-altering diagnosis. The realization of the loss is the main foundation for the depression. A recent study suggests that 35% of newly diagnosed AD clients become depressed.
- Clients need to be around people and participate in activities. The activities need to be appropriate for their cognitive level. Making the task too difficult causes an undesired effect. Encourage clients to help set the table before dinner or get the checkbook to help with paying the bills.
- Without treatment, postdiagnosis depression can cause rapid cognitive decline.
- Depression produces feelings of hopelessness, sadness, and crying. Difficulty in concentrating, the loss of sleep, and a decline in appetite and weight occur frequently.
- Depressed people commonly use alcohol and tranquilizers to self-medicate. Because the depression decreases clients' ability to function, the cognitive impairment inhibits the client's ability to control self-medicating or drinking.
- Encourage friends to visit and talk to clients while maintaining eye contact and keeping them involved in the conversation. Sometimes talking to a qualified counselor or clergy can help with the feeling of sorrow.

Apathy

- Apathy, indifference, and lethargy are commonly seen in AD clients. A lack of interest and initiative hinders their ability to participate in activities.
- Communication and activity with the client help relieve feelings of apathy. Activity is important, both physically and psychologically. An unexercised mind is just as dangerous as an unexercised body.
- Encourage participation in group activities.
- Forcing a person to join an activity may make the person feel anxious, scared, and agitated. Small accomplishments should be praised.

Anxiety

- Anxiety, restlessness, and nervousness commonly accompany AD. Anxiety elicits behaviors that may at times be irritating to others.

- Repetitive behaviors of pacing or fidgeting may be the outcome of the client's inability to verbalize.
- Remember the client is not doing this on purpose; the behavior is the result of the brain dysfunction.

Lecture Material for Slide 7-9

LEGAL ISSUES

Everyone with AD progresses at a different rate. Unfortunately, clients become incapable of making medical and legal decisions for themselves. The diagnosis of Alzheimer's brings about important and difficult issues. Clients need to participate in planning for their future before they become incompetent or their wishes may not be executed.

Guardianship

Guardianship, or conservatorship, is a legal process used when an individual no longer can make or communicate appropriate or sound decisions about his or her person and/or property. If decisions are not made while the client is still of sound mind and body, a court-appointed guardian is assigned.

Durable Power of Attorney (DPA)

The DPA establishes a legal relationship between the client and an appointed person or agent to serve as a substitute decision maker. The term "durable" indicates the decision making remains in effect after the incapacity of the person.

- A DPA for health care identifies an agent to make all health-related decisions including end-of-life care.
- A DPA for property identifies an agent to control income and assets only.

Last Will and Testament

A last will and testament is a legal document providing for the distribution of a person's property and assets after death. Without a will, the client's estate is distributed according to state law.

Living Will

A living will is a document stating the client's end-of-life wishes. This document does not account for all health care decisions.

Advanced Directive

The Patient Self-Determination Act of 1990 mandates health care providers to furnish information regarding advanced directives. An advanced directive is a legal document describing the client's wishes regarding supportive or life-sustaining treatments.

Lecture Material for Slide 7-10

CARE OPTIONS

Caring for a family member with AD is difficult, stressful, and disruptive to the home. Many different types of help are available. The choice of the support chosen is dependent on the family's needs.

Home Care

Home care is an in-home service provided by a qualified agency to support the medical needs of a client in the home. Services range from basic housekeeping duties to physician visits.

- The home care aide (HCA) helps with home tasks, such as laundry, meal preparation, house cleaning, and food shopping. Removing these responsibilities from the family allows them to spend quality and priceless time with their loved one.
- The home care aide also assists the client with daily care, including bathing, dressing, and feeding. Assistance with daily care needs helps the family with the heavy and physically challenging aspect of personal care. In most cases the spouse is elderly and is unable to perform custodial care.

Respite Care

Respite care is temporary help for families caring for those with disabilities, chronic or terminal illnesses, and the elderly. Relief may come in the form of a sitter, friend, or HCA, who provides the caregiver with personal time away from the client.

- Frequently, the family is expending all their free time and energy caring for their loved one. Everyone needs personal and recreation time to take care of individual needs and family obligations.
- A family member may feel guilty needing time away from the loved one. "Dad won't be around forever. What is wrong with me?" Needing time away from a stressful situation is natural and warranted. Caregivers experiencing work overload and interpersonal conflict over an extended period of time are more prone to burnout.
- Caregiver burnout has serious impacts on the person, the client, and the health care team. Clients may receive a lower quality of care due to the caregiver's fatigue.

Adult Day Care

Adult day care provides another form of respite care as well as socialization for the client. The daily service, consisting of several hours, offers activities, limited medical care, and companionship. Although clients may be unable to perform previous activities, they are able to enjoy music, pet therapy, and singing.

Assisted Living

Assisted living is a state-regulated, residential, long-term care alternative. Assisted living coordinates services to meet the needs of residents based on assessments and service plans. The living arrangement allows for independence with assistance. As the client's condition declines, the use of services is increased based on needs.

Long-Term Care Facilities (LTC)

LTC facilities provide 24-hour nursing supervision for the client. The facility can provide medical interventions including intravenous therapy, rehabilitation care, ventilator-dependent care, and custodial care. Nursing home placement should be thoroughly discussed with all parties involved before the decision has to be made.

SUMMING UP

The affects of AD extend far beyond the client's physical and mental requirements. The family and the AD client all experience changes in the roles and responsibilities of the family unit. A wife, child, or husband now is forced to become the breadwinner, parent, and caregiver. Although everyone responds to loss and grief differently and has his or her own way of handling stress, the feelings experienced are very similar.

Physical and financial care needs should be addressed prior to the AD clients becoming unable to assist with the decision-making. Many different types of care and protection exist. The client and family need to review all options as soon as the diagnosis is conveyed.

The AD client perceives his or her illness differently from how a healthy person may think of the illness. Perhaps society needs education and insight into the disease. The AD client's current abilities need to be nurtured and cherished to make the most of the situation. Focus on the here and now and treasure every day.

Instructor's Version with Answers to Handout 7-2

● REAL-LIFE SCENARIO

A Day in the Life of Pat

Pat is a schoolteacher and is experiencing difficulty remembering students' names, lesson plans, and after-school meetings. Pat's family and colleagues are noticing personality and performance changes. Pat's family encourages a visit to the physician. Following a diagnostic evaluation, Pat is diagnosed with AD.

1. With the diagnosis of AD come changes in role. List five factors affecting role.

   Factors affecting role include environment, leadership, responsibility, socializing, and role reversal.

2. Name the stages of grief defined by Dr. Elisabeth Kubler-Ross.

   The stages of grief as defined by Dr. Elisabeth Kubler-Ross are denial and isolation, anger, bargaining, depression, and acceptance.

3. List common emotions experienced by the client with Alzheimer's disease.

   Common emotions experienced with AD are depression, apathy, and anxiety.

4. What legal issues should Pat explore, in the early stage of the disease, to avoid having a court-appointed guardian?

   Pat should explore the following legal issues when in the early stage of the disease: durable power of attorney, last will and testament, a living will or an advance directive.

GROUP ACTIVITY

● PURPOSE OF THE ACTIVITY

The purpose of this activity is to explore personal feelings regarding a diagnosis of AD. The following activity can be completed as a class, in small groups, or individually.

Instruct the students to list their current roles and explain how a diagnosis of dementia would affect those roles. Continue the exercise by including how their roles would change if a family member were diagnosed with the disease. Discuss all answers.

Name _____ Date _____

Program/Course _____ Instructor's Name _____

Coping with Dementia Pre- and Post-Test

1. How does Alzheimer's disease affect individuals, families, caregivers, and society?
   a. Alzheimer's disease changes roles.
   b. Alzheimer's disease impacts finances.
   c. Alzheimer's disease causes caregivers to learn basic nursing skills.
   d. All of the above.

2. Which is *not* a common emotion felt by a client with dementia?
   a. Depression
   b. Jealousy
   c. Apathy
   d. Fear

3. When should end-of-life care decisions be discussed with newly diagnosed clients?
   a. When they are at the end of the disease process.
   b. When they are in a nursing home.
   c. When they are first diagnosed and capable of making decisions.
   d. Whenever the family feels ready to make the decision.

4. List the stages of grief according to Elisabeth Kubler-Ross.
   a. Denial and isolation, anger, bargaining, depression, acceptance.
   b. Isolation, anger, bargaining and depression, adaptation.
   c. Denial, isolation, depression, bartering, hopelessness.
   d. Denial and isolation, apathy, bargaining, depression, adaptation.

5. What is a durable power of attorney?
   a. An appointed person who makes financial and/or health care decisions for a person who is incompetent.
   b. An appointed person who assists families with decision making.
   c. A document stating the end-of-life wishes for the client.
   d. A document that describes the distribution of personal property.

Handout **7-1**

A Day in the Life of Pat: A Real-Life Scenario

Pat is a schoolteacher and is experiencing difficulty remembering students' names, lesson plans, and after-school meetings. Pat's family and colleagues are noticing personality and performance changes. Pat's family encourages a visit to the physician. Following a diagnostic evaluation, Pat is diagnosed with AD.

1. With the diagnosis of AD come changes in role. List five factors affecting role.

2. Name the stages of grief defined by Dr. Elisabeth Kubler-Ross.

3. List common emotions experienced by the client with Alzheimer's disease.

4. What legal issues should Pat explore, in the early stage of the disease, to avoid having a court-appointed guardian?

Handout 7-2

MODULE 7 COPYING WITH DEMENTIA

Transparency Master **7-1**

Early in the Disease Process

- **Trivialize the memory loss**
- **Unaware of the progressing condition**
- **Varying perception of symptoms**
- **Concerns about making mistakes**

Early in the Disease Process (cont.)

- **Suspicion, loneliness and fear**
- **Impact on social activities**
- **Live in the here and now**

Changes Affecting Role

- **Environment**
- **Leadership**
- **Responsibility**
- **Socializing**
- **Role reversal**

When the Client Is a Parent

- **Role reversal**
- **Lack of confidence in new role**
- **Feelings of loss**

When the Client Is a Spouse

- **Transition of leadership**
- **Absorption of new responsibilities**
- **Overwhelmed with emotion**

Stages of Grief

- **Denial and isolation**
- **Anger**
- **Bargaining**
- **Depression**
- **Acceptance**

Emotions of Dementia

- **Depression**
- **Apathy**
- **Anxiety**

Legal Issues

- Guardianship
- Durable power of attorney (DPA)
- Last will and testament
- Living will
- Advanced directive

Care Options

- **Homecare**
- **Respite care**
- **Adult day care**
- **Assisted living**
- **Long-term care facilities (LTC)**

Module 8
Caring for the Caregiver

Goal
To educate the caregiver on the importance of maintaining a healthy and supportive environment.

Objectives
After the completion of the presentation, students will be able to:

- Discuss the burdens of caregiving and caregiver burnout.
- Define the terms "informal caregiver" and "formal caregiver."
- List five signs and symptoms of burnout.
- Explain four techniques to reduce stress.
- Describe how the dementia client is at an increased risk for elder abuse.
- List the three categories of elder abuse.

GENERAL INFORMATION/OVERVIEW

Lecture Material for Slide 8-1

Caregiving is stressful and labor-intensive. In a recent study, symptoms of stress, depression, and chronic immunosuppression were found to be three times more common in caregivers when compared to noncaregivers.

Caregivers often have unpleasant duties, such as emptying bedpans and changing soiled bed linens. Clients may be disoriented, irritable, or uncooperative. The caregiver role has dangers including caring for clients whose illness may cause violent behavior or exposure to an infectious disease. While the work can be emotionally demanding, many caregivers gain satisfaction from assisting others in times of need.

Studies on stress in the health care field have attempted to measure the effects of stress on health and well-being. Work-related stress can affect job satisfaction and mental health. Stress may also contribute to some forms of physical illness, particularly musculoskeletal problems.

- The most stressful reported aspect of caregiving is caring for the incontinent and/or dementia client. Personal care tasks, such as bathing, are also reported as being laborious.
- Caregivers assisting Alzheimer's clients reported three times as many emotional stress symptoms as the general population.
- Caregivers report stressors are related to time restrictions and limited social interaction.
- The levels of support given by other informal or formal caregivers affect overall satisfaction.
- Health care workers are exposed to a high rate of violent behavior.
- Symptoms of depression, anxiety, helplessness, isolation, low morale, and emotional exhaustion are commonly reported by caregivers.
- Many caregivers have health and family problems in addition to the illness of their clients, friends, or family members.

BURDENS OF CAREGIVING AND CAREGIVER BURNOUT

Lecture Material for Slide 8-2

The impact of caregiving is evaluated by examining how caregiving disrupts daily routines, social relationships, perceptions, and reactions to demands.

- "Caregiver burden" is an industry term used to define the physical, emotional, financial, and social problems associated with caregiving.
- Stressors erode the caregiver's mental and physical health. Caregiver burnout is the direct result of stress. Caregivers experiencing work overload and interpersonal conflict over an extended period of time are more sensitive to burnout.
- Caregiver burnout has serious impacts on the person, the client, and the health care team. Clients may receive a lower quality of care due

to the caregiver's fatigue. The caregiver may become less sensitive to the client's feelings and become detached from the environment. If the burnout continues without intervention, frequent tardiness or absenteeism may result.

- The early warning signs of burnout may include feeling less motivated, working additional hours with fewer results, and complaining about the caregiving role. The caregiver carries these feelings home and to the work environment, therefore limiting meaningful interactions. Physical, psychological, and behavioral changes can be observed in the later stages of burnout.
- Both formal and informal caregivers can develop caregiver burden or burnout.

Lecture Material for Slide 8-3

INFORMAL CAREGIVERS

Informal caregivers are individuals who voluntarily provide care without pay, formal education, and training. Informal caregivers include immediate family members such as spouses, children, brothers, sisters, and other relatives of the client. Friends, neighbors, and volunteers from churches, charities, and community groups can also be informal caregivers.

- During any given year, more than 50 million people provide care for the chronically ill, disabled, aged family member or friend. (National Family Caregivers Association, 2006)
- Informal caregivers are reluctant to use the term "caregivers" since the label is associated with compensation. Most families feel their participation in the care of a family member is "what families do" and feel the caregiver role is separate.
- Individuals who identify themselves as caregivers are providing complete care to their loved ones.
- Since family caregivers feel their acquired tasks are part of the family dynamics, many are hesitant to complain about the role.
- The typical caregiver is a daughter, age 46, with a full-time job, providing an average of 18 hours per week to one or both parents.
- Forty-four percent of the caregiving population is male. (National Family Caregivers Association, 2005)
- Among adults aged 20 to 75, 38% care for aging parents and 11% care for their spouses.
- Appropriately 45% of working caregivers report having to rearrange work schedules, decrease work hours, or take an unpaid leave to meet their caregiving responsibilities.
- A recent study estimates informal caregivers lose approximately $660,000 in wages over their lifetime because of missed work.
- Productivity losses to businesses because of employees missing work for caregiving responsibilities range from $11 to $29 billion annually.

- The average time informal caregivers provide assistance is four and a half years, but 20% provide care for five years or longer.
- The stress of family caregiving for people with dementia has shown to impact a caregiver's immune system for up to three years after their caregiving ends; thus increasing their chances of developing a chronic illness themselves.

Causes of Burden for Informal Caregivers

- Unexpected changes in a preexisting role and social activities
- Physical demands (being on-call 24 hours a day)
- Having to learn basic nursing skills
- The emotional issues of caring for someone with a terminal illness
- Financial impact

Lecture Material for Slide 8-4

FORMAL CAREGIVERS

Formal caregivers are volunteers or paid care providers associated with an organization who provide care as a profession or an occupation. Formal caregivers include physicians, nurses, and licensed and nonlicensed personnel. Formal caregivers may work in nursing homes, intermediate care facilities, assisted living facilities, home care agencies, community services, hospice, churches, charity service groups, adult day care centers, senior centers, or state aging services.

- Personal care assistants and home care aides occupied 701,000 U.S. jobs in 2004. Nurses aides, psychiatric aides, and home health aides held more than two million U.S. jobs in 2004. Nurses aides held 1.4 million of those positions. (Bureau of Labor Statistics, 2006)
- Two out of five nurses aides work in facilities and one quarter work in hospitals. (Bureau of Labor Statistics, 2005)
- According to the Health Care Financing Administration, more than 20,000 providers deliver home care services to 7.6 million individuals due to acute illness, long-term health conditions, permanent disability, or terminal illness. (NAHC)
- The role of a formal caregiver is associated with multiple and conflicting demands imposed by nurse supervisors, managers, medical and administrative staff, clients, and families. The requirements appear to lead to work overload and role conflict.
- Nursing aides employed in nursing care facilities often are the principal caregivers, having far more contact with residents than other members of the staff. Because some residents may stay in a nursing care facility for months or even years, aides develop ongoing relationships with clients and interact with them positively and caringly.

Causes of Burden for Formal Caregivers

Formal caregivers:

- Have similar burdens to those of informal caregivers.
- May experience a lack of support from their families and professional co-workers.
- Experience workplace-related stressors (work overload, unrealistic expectations, lack of decision-making autonomy, communication problems, and inadequate medical resources).

THE EFFECTS OF CAREGIVER BURDEN

The numerous duties performed by caregivers leave little personal time. Most neglect their own health. Caregivers are less likely to eat well-balanced meals, exercise regularly, and participate in stress-management or health-promotion activities.

- Performing the actual tasks of caregiving, as well as the number and intensity of each activity, has a profound affect on individuals.
- The signs and symptoms of caregiver burden can differ for each individual. The extent of symptoms depends on the personalities, belief systems, general health, energy levels, and coping skills.
- The severity of the client's condition, the duration of caregiving, and support systems are also factors affecting caregiver burden.

Assistance Needed in Long-Term Care

Residents of long-term care facilities customarily have multiple co-morbid conditions. The level of assistance each client requires greatly impacts the effects of caregiver burden. The following accounts for the percentage of residence requiring assistance with personal care needs:

- 96.2 percent need assistance with bathing or showering.
- 87.2 percent need assistance with dressing.
- 56.2 percent need assistance with toileting.
- 45 percent need assistance with eating.
- 25.4 percent need assistance with transfers.

STRESS

Stress is the result of everyday responsibilities, obligations, and pressures. Everyone experiences stress differently, but the cause is always related to a negative feeling (being late for work or losing a job). Unfortunately, in society, no quick and easy cure has been discovered to alleviate stress.

In response to daily (physiological) stress, the body automatically increases:
- Blood pressure.
- Heart and respiratory rate.
- Metabolism.
- Blood flow to muscles.

Physical stress is caused by:
- Doing too much.
- Illness.
- Inadequate sleep.
- Poor diet.

Emotional stress may lead to:
- Anger and frustration.
- Low self-esteem.
- Feelings of helplessness.
- Mood swings.

Emotional stress is triggered by:
- Money problems.
- Illness.
- Family and friends.
- Life changes.

Audience Interaction for Slide 8-6

Ask the audience for the common signs and symptoms of burnout. Include the following in the discussion. Use Handout 8-2 as the guide. The following table can be used in the discussion.

Physical Signs	Psychological Signs	Behavioral Signs
Backaches	Anger and frustration	Emotional outbursts
Changes in eating habits	Decreased self-confidence and self-esteem	Withdrawal from friends and family
Elevated blood pressure	Loss of interest in hobbies and work	Loss of punctuality and neglect of duty
Fatigue	Feelings of inadequacy, helplessness	Decrease in judgment
Gastrointestinal problems	Feelings of restlessness	Inability to focus on tasks
Headaches	Depression	Tearfulness
Insomnia	Sense of being overwhelmed or overloaded	Increased use of chemical substances
Muscle tension	Mood swings	Difficulty getting along with others
Weight loss	Sense of failure / Anxiety about future	Impaired work performance / Resistance to change

(O'Neill and McKinney, 2003)

Ask the audience to list the rewards of caregiving. Possible answers may include:

- Brings meaning and purpose to one's life.
- Empathy and understanding.
- Sense of personal pride in handling difficult circumstances.
- Positive feelings associated with being needed.

Lecture Material for Slides 8-7 and 8-8

Slide 8-7

CONQUERING THE EFFECTS OF CAREGIVER BURDEN AND BURNOUT

Insert agency's policies and support systems to assist employees with caregiver burden and burnout.

The most effective strategy in reducing the effects of caregiver burden and burnout is to manage the environment. Develop a plan and continually reevaluate the environment to reduce unnecessary burdens. Incorporate support groups or regular case discussions into the plan. The discussions should advocate training, information sharing, and comprehensive approaches to care. Creating an open forum for formal caregivers allows them to share coping patterns, solutions to workplace issues, and improvements for overall job satisfaction.

Problem-Solving Approach to Reduce Caregiver Burden/Burnout

Problem-solving techniques involve gathering information and identifying the issues, causes, and alternatives to a problem. Very often defining the problem is more arduous than discovering the solution. Exploring all aspects of the dilemma may alleviate some aspects of the problem.

The Problem-Solving Approach

- Define the overall needs, purposes, and goals.
- Define the problems.
- Analyze strengths and weakness.
- Determine available resources.
- Reevaluate demands, reducing or eliminating excessive demands.

Slide 8-8

- Set priorities.
- Generate solutions.
- Implement solutions.
- Incorporate techniques to reduce stress.
- Discuss concerns with the supervisor or other members of the facility, family, friends, or physician.
- Evaluate the effectiveness of change.

Audience Interaction for Slides 8-7 and 8-8

Ask the audience what interventions should be taken following a stressful situation with a client or family member? Discuss the answers.

Possible answers are:

- Notify the supervisor.
- Do not argue. (This only increases the stress.)
- Provide safety for the client.
- Step away from the situation. (Being away from the situation allows for better perception of the issue.)
- Perform relaxation exercises (deep breathing or counting).
- Leave the area.

Lecture Material for Slides 8-9 and 8-10

Slide 8-9

TECHNIQUES TO REDUCE STRESS

The key to stress management is balance. When dealing with stress, determine a personal tolerance level and attempt to live within the limits. Stress cannot be completely eliminated; instead, learn to manage stressful situations.

Time Management

- A person who uses time efficiently generally experiences less stress related to family and job activities.
- Learn to say no to tasks that do not fit into the schedule.
- Schedule appointments realistically. Organizing the day eliminates the need to rush from task to task or errand to errand.
- Controlling the demands of others is essential for effective time management. Few people are able to meet all the requests made by others. Learn to recognize which requests can be realistically met. Determine if any of the requests are negotiable.
- Make a list and check off each item when completed. This provides a positive feeling of accomplishment. Organize the day effectively; use an appointment book or calendar to plan.

Forget the Superhero Image

- Learn to compromise.
- Set priorities and realistic goals.
- Eliminate unnecessary activities. Do not take on more than can be handled.
- No one is perfect.
- Ask for help.
- Set limits.
- Delegate work.

Ways to Ask for Help

- Set aside time to talk to an individual who can help.
- Review the lists of client needs.
- Discuss specific areas where the individual can help; then ask.
- Verify that the individual fully understands exactly what should be done. Do not assume the individual knows what will help. Explain the tasks.

Use Relaxation Techniques

- Relaxation techniques are methods, such as deep breathing, that allow a person to relax.
- To relax, learn to recognize the stress.
- Attempt meditation or quiet time (taking a bath, listening to music, sitting in a dark room).
- Visualization (think "happy thoughts") enhances self-confidence and makes an upcoming stressful event easier to manage.

Exercise

- Twenty-eight percent of Americans live a sedentary lifestyle.
- Exercise helps the body to function optimally.
- A decrease in physical activity is a risk factor for heart disease, diabetes mellitus, colon cancer, hypertension, obesity, osteoporosis, muscle and joint disorders, as well as early death.
- Regular exercise improves muscle and bone strength, also improving endurance.
- Exercise helps control blood glucose, cholesterol levels, and weight. Anxiety and depression may be reduced with physical activity.
- Exercise increases HDL (good fats) in the blood.
- According to the Centers for Disease Control and Prevention (CDC), walking qualifies as moderate-intensity aerobic activity. Participation in an accumulated 30 minutes of moderate-level daily physical activity is recommended.
- Routine exercise should began in early school years and continue throughout a lifetime.

Slide 8-10

Choose a Favorite Activity

Maintain a life outside of the caregiver role. The burden of caring for others may cause neglect to friends, family, or other activities once enjoyed.

- Take up a new hobby.
- Relax in a worry-free environment.
- Indulge with music, bubble baths, watching a sunset.
- Create personal time.

Talk to Others and Use Support Systems

- A support system of family, friends, and coworkers who will listen, offer advice, and emotional support is beneficial to a stressed individual.
- Support systems can reduce stress reactions, as well as promote physical and mental well-being.

Be Flexible

- An individual's perception of stress plays a major role in the ability to cope and remain flexible in an adverse situation.
- Flexibility promotes the most appropriate action for the situation. Maintaining efficiency in a stressful situation does not require giving in or avoiding a stressor.
- Put things in perspective; some situations are not worth worrying or fighting about. Pick the battles.

Audience Interaction for Slide 8-11

"Healthy living" is a term with a multitude of interpretations. Ask the audience to define the term "healthy living" and discuss the answers.

Lecture Material for Slide 8-11

● HEALTHY LIVING

Healthy eating, getting enough sleep, daily exercise, and avoiding high-risk behaviors are part of a healthy lifestyle. A healthy body adapts better to stressful situations.

Diet

- Follow the recommended dietary guidelines. Eat more fruits and vegetables. Choose foods low in saturated fats.
- Unsaturated fats (canola oil, olive oil, corn oil) help protect against heart disease and lower LDL levels (bad fats). Saturated fats (eg, butter, Crisco®) increase cholesterol levels.
- Tobacco use, a poor diet, and the lack of exercise are major risk factors for death.
- Poor eating habits are learned in childhood and carried through adulthood.
- On average, less than one fourth of American adults consume the recommended amounts of fruits and vegetables.
- Thirty percent of cancer deaths are the result of dietary risk factors.
- Poor diet increases risks of chronic illnesses, including diabetes mellitus, cancer, and heart disease.

Rest

- Adequate rest can be considered a preventive measure. Insufficient restful sleep can cause health problems. Sleep is an active state that affects both physical and mental well-being.

- One study demonstrates sleep deprivation has dramatic effects on the brain and its performance. The brain works harder and accomplishes less when tired.
- Busy schedules can result in less than adequate sleep. Eight hours of sleep a night is recommended.

Tobacco

- Cigarette smoking is the leading cause of premature death in the United States.
- The Surgeon General has called tobacco smoke "the most important of the known modifiable risk factors for coronary heart disease."
- Smoking is a major risk factor leading to four of the five foremost causes of death, including heart attack, stroke, cancer, and lung disease.
- Smoking decreases the ratio of HDL (good fats) to LDL (bad fats), increasing the risk of coronary heart disease.
- Smoking acts synergistically with other risk factors for coronary artery disease.

Lecture Material for Slide 8-12

● REDUCING RISK FACTORS

Risk factors are conditions causing a person to become particularly vulnerable to an unwanted event. The more risk factors a person has, the greater the likelihood is of developing a disease. For some conditions, one or more risk factors have a synergistic effect.

Nonmodifiable Risk Factors

Nonmodifiable risk factors are conditions that cannot be altered or changed. Determining nonmodifiable risk factors enables the person to make better options concerning controllable lifestyle choices.

Nonmodifiable risk factors are:
- Heredity.
- Gender.
- Race.
- Age.

Modifiable Risk Factors

Modifiable risk factors are risk factors that can be changed by the individual. Risk factors that can be changed directly influence the occurrence of chronic diseases.

Modifiable risk factors are:
- Tobacco use.
- Drug and alcohol use.
- Hypertension.
- Blood cholesterol levels.
- Diet.
- Obesity.
- Physical inactivity.
- Sexual promiscuity.

Lecture Material for Slide 8-13

STRESS AND ELDER ABUSE

The stress of caring for the older adult is a significant risk factor for abuse and neglect. Caregivers experience intense frustration and anger. In the absence of proper management skills, the frustration may lead to a range of abusive behaviors. The demands of caregiving are never fully understood until personally experienced.

- The risk of abuse increases as the client's disabilities worsen.
- Most caregivers do not have appropriate training. If not properly trained for dealing with difficult behaviors, caregivers can find themselves using physical force.
- Preventing elder abuse is learning how to balance the needs of the older adult with the caregiver's own needs.
- The lack of available resources and assistance may increase the stress level of the caregiver.
- For every case of elder abuse and neglect that is reported, experts believe there may be five cases not reported.
- Elders who are ill, frail, disabled, mentally impaired, or depressed are at greater risk of abuse.
- Clients 80 years and older are two to three times more likely to be abused or neglected than the remaining elderly population.
- Older adults who have been abused tend to die sooner than those who are not abused, even in the absence of disease.

Federal Laws

Federal definitions of elder abuse, neglect, and exploitation appeared for the first time in the 1987 Amendments to the Older Americans Act (42 U.S.C. 3001 et seq., as amended). This amendment provides guidelines for identifying problems of elder abuse; the amendment has no enforcement purpose. The Older Americans Act established the Long-Term Care Ombudsman in 1972, to address the mistreatment of residents. The Ombudsman office serves as advocates for residents of long-term care facilities. The Ombudsman's office investigates complaints by visiting with residents, resident's family, staff, and administrators of the facility, and possibly adult protective services and law enforcement agencies.

- In 2003, state long-term care Ombudsman programs nationally investigated over 226,000 complaints of abuse, gross neglect, and exploitation on behalf of residents. Among seven types of abuse categories, physical abuse was the most common type reported. (Administration on Aging, 2005)
- State laws and definitions of elder abuse vary in what constitutes abuse, neglect, or exploitation of the elderly.
- Presently, no federal laws for elder abuse exist that are equivalent to the federal laws on child abuse.

Contact the local office on aging for more information regarding specific state definitions and requirements. The National Center on Elder Abuse (NCEA) can provide individual state information (www.elderabusecenter.org).

● CATEGORIES OF ELDER ABUSE

Lecture Material for Slide 8-14

The categories of abuse are domestic abuse, institutional abuse, and self-neglect. The elderly are living longer and are dependent on others for care.

Domestic Elder Abuse

Domestic elder abuse is any form of maltreatment of an older person by someone, who has a special relationship with the elder (spouse, child, friend, or caregiver) or who is living in the older person's own home or in the home of a caregiver. This form of abuse includes physical, emotional, sexual, neglect, and abandonment.

Institutional Elder Abuse

Institutional elder abuse refers to any form of abuse that occurs in residential facilities, nursing homes, foster homes, group homes, or board and care. The abusers can be any persons who have a legal or contractual obligation to provide the elderly with care and protection (paid caregivers, staff, professionals).

Self-Neglect or Self-Abuse

Self-neglect or abuse includes any behavior or action by an elder that threatens his or her own health or safety, even if due to their physical or psychological limitations.

Lecture Material for Slide 8-15

TYPES OF ABUSE

Elder abuse can take a number of different forms and may be defined in varying ways. Even if the senior is not in a high risk group they can find themselves in abusive situations.

Physical Abuse

Physical abuse is the use of physical force resulting in bodily injury, pain, or physical impairment. Examples of physical abuse are hitting, shoving, shaking, slapping, kicking, pinching, burning, inappropriate use of restraints (physical or chemical restraints or sedation), or force-feeding.

Signs of Physical Abuse

- Change in the client's overall appearance
- Sudden changes in the client's behavior not due to illness or medication
- Bruises, especially where covered by clothing
- Blackeyes and broken eyeglasses or frames
- Fractures
- Cuts, lacerations, and welts
- Untreated injuries in various stages of healing
- Sprains and dislocations
- Internal injuries and bleeding
- Signs of being restrained (rope burns)

Emotional/Physiological Abuse

Emotional abuse is mental or emotional distress through verbal or nonverbal acts, including humiliation, intimidation, or harassment. The abuse isolates the elderly person from his or her family, friends, or regular activities.

Signs of Emotional Abuse

- Being emotionally upset or agitated
- Being withdrawn, uncommunicative, or unresponsive
- Difficulty sleeping
- Unusual behavior such as sucking, biting, or rocking
- Improvement of behavior when not in the care of the abuser

Sexual Abuse

Sexual abuse is the nonconsensual sexual contact of any kind or sexual contacts with any person incapable of giving their consent. Also included are unwanted touching, all types of sexual assault and/or battery, coerced nudity, and sexually explicit photography.

Signs of Sexual Abuse
- Injuries around the breasts or genital area
- Venereal disease without explanation
- Vaginal or anal bleeding without explanation
- Torn, stained, or bloody undergarments
- Pain when walking or sitting

Financial Abuse

Financial abuse is stealing or misusing money or property, for someone else's benefit, without the older adult's knowledge. Examples of financial abuse are:
- Cashing the person's checks without their permission.
- Forging their signature.
- Misusing their money or possessions.
- Coercing or deceiving an older person into signing a document (contracts or will).
- Misuse of a guardianship or power of attorney.

Signs of Financial Abuse
- Bank account changes
- Unexplained transfers of assets to a family member or someone outside the family
- Unexplained withdrawals of large sums of money
- Additional names on bank accounts
- Unauthorized withdrawals of funds using the ATM card
- Forged signatures for financial transactions or for the titles of possessions
- Changes in the will
- Bills unpaid despite ample financial resources
- Payment for services that are not necessary (such as a lawn service for a client living in an apartment)
- Valuables disappearing from the client's home
- Uninvolved relatives claiming rights to the client's possessions

Neglect

Neglect, the most common form of elder maltreatment, is the refusal or failure of a caregiver to provide the basic needs to the elder, including food, clothing, shelter, and medical care.
- Failure to provide the services necessary to avoid physical harm, mental anguish, and home safety.

- Failure of the person with fiduciary responsibilities to provide care for the older client. The person with power of attorney refuses to pay for the necessary home care services.
- Failure of a paid in-home service provider to arrange the necessary care. An example is when a HCA does not go to the scheduled case.

Signs of Neglect

- Dehydration
- Malnutrition
- Inappropriate dress for weather conditions
- Caregiver's refusal of visitors
- Untreated pressure ulcers
- Poor personal hygiene
- Untreated health problems
- Hazardous or unsafe living conditions or arrangements
- Improper electrical wiring, no heat or running water
- An unsanitary living condition, such as dirt, flees, or soiled bedding

Self-Neglect

Self-neglect includes any behavior or action that threatens an older person's health or safety, and arises from his or her physical or psychological limitations. Many elderly are isolated, contributing to the neglect.

- The definition of self-neglect *excludes* a client who is mentally competent and understands the consequences of his or her decisions. No one can force competent adults to change the way they live even if their actions can threaten their health or safety. The elderly have the right to determine their affairs to the full extent of their ability as long as they are deemed competent.
- The client may refuse or fail to provide him or herself with adequate food, water, clothing, shelter, personal hygiene, medication, and safety precautions.
- Most cases of self-neglect are by women.
- Forty-five percent of self-neglect cases involve people over the age of 80.

Signs of Self-Neglect

- The inability to manage personal finances, failing to pay bills, stashing money, or giving money away.
- The inability to maintain activities of daily living, including personal care, food shopping, meal preparation, housekeeping, and inadequate clothing.
- The inability to maintain safety, as exhibited by wanderings, refusing medical attention, leaving the stove on, and/or a lack of security.

- An unsafe living environment: no utilities, no working toilets, faulty wiring, or even homelessness.
- Declining health status with dehydration, malnutrition, and untreated illnesses.
- Changes in mental status with confusion, inappropriate responses, disorientation, and memory loss.
- Lack of medical interventions such as eyeglasses, hearing aides, dentures, DME, and missed doctor's appointments.

Abandonment

Abandonment, a form of neglect, occurs when the caregiver leaves the elderly person with no intention of resuming the caregiver role.

- The elderly person may be left at a health care facility (hospital, nursing home, adult day care center), and the caregiver refuses to pick the client up at the time of discharge or is unable to be reached or contacted. The caregiver may also "dump" the client at the emergency department of the hospital and not return.
- The elder may also be left in a public location (a shopping center, library, parking lot, bus station), and the caregiver no longer wants to accept responsibility for the client. The elderly person may be confused and unable to identify the caregiver or their residence.

WHO ABUSES

Abusers of the elderly can be women or men. Family members are more often the abusers. In previous years, data reported adult children were the most common abusers of the elderly as compared to other family members. Recent information indicates spouses may be more commonly the perpetrators. The abuser can also be an informal or formal caregiver.

Indicators of Abuse by the Caregiver

The abuser may exhibit warning signs when the older adult is in the presence of others. The caregiver or abuser may:

- Prevent the older adult to speak for him or herself.
- Be apathetic or angry toward the elderly person.
- Fail to assist the older adult.
- Blame the client for accidents, accusing the older person of deliberately spilling food or soiling the bed.
- Exhibit aggressive behaviors (threats, insults, and harassment) toward the elderly person.
- Be overly affectionate around company or outsiders.
- Display inappropriate sexual behavior with the older adult.

- Restrict activities or isolate the client from family (sometimes threatening to keep people away from the older person because isolation increases the probability of abuse).
- Have contradictory versions of events concerning the elder adult.
- Be non-compliant with service providers in planning care.
- Be very defensive when approached about the elder.

Reporting Elder Abuse

Each state designates who is mandated to report incidences of elder abuse. The Adult Protective Services (APS) is the principal public agency responsible both for investigating reported cases of elder abuse and for providing victims and their families with treatment and protective services.

Contact the local Adult Protective Services for individual state information.

Insert agency policy regarding reporting abuse here.

SUMMING UP

Caregiving is a stressful undertaking, many times leading to caregiver burden or burnout. The stress of being a caregiver causes unexpected changes in roles and social activities. The responsibility has many physical demands, often requiring the caregiver to learn new skills and possibly having a financial impact. Caregiving requires learning problem-solving techniques. The caregiver needs to determine the goals, find resources, and analyze strengths and weaknesses.

Many techniques exist for reducing stress. The techniques should be identified and utilized to prevent burnout. Eating well, getting adequate rest, and reducing the use of tobacco can help caregivers reduce their risk for illness. Elder abuse exists and is often the result of caregiver burnout or depression.

Instructor's Version with Answers to Handout 8-4

● REAL-LIFE SCENARIO

A Day in the Life of Pat

Pat is a schoolteacher and has an elderly father with dementia. Since Pat's mom is deceased, the only option was to move Pat's father to live with Pat. Upon Pat's arrival home, water is flowing from the kitchen faucet, over the countertop, and onto the floor. Dad was found on the flooded kitchen floor, soiled. Pat becomes enraged and demoralizes him by yelling and screaming obscenities and insults.

1. List the possible causes for Pat's caregiver burden.

   Physical demands.

   Unexpected role change.

   Unexpected living conditions.

   Financial impact.

   Emotional stress of caring for an ill parent.

2. Describe the problem-solving approache to help reduce caregiver burden.
   - *Define the overall needs and goal.*
   - *Define the problem.*
   - *Determine the available resources.*
   - *Reduce excessive demands.*
   - *Set priorities.*
   - *Generate solutions.*
   - *Implement solutions.*
   - *Incorporate techniques to reduce stress.*
   - *Discuss concerns with the supervisor.*

3. Describe five types of abuse observed with the elderly. What types of abuse are noted in the scenario?
   - *Physical abuse is the use of physical force resulting in bodily injury, pain, or physical impairment.*
   - *Emotional abuse is mental or emotional distress through verbal or nonverbal acts, including humiliation, intimidation, or harassment.*
   - *Sexual abuse is the nonconsensual sexual contact of any kind or sexual contacts with any person incapable of giving consent.*
   - *Neglect, the most common form of elder maltreatment, is the refusal or failure of a caregiver to provide the basic needs to the elder, including food, clothing, shelter, and medical care.*
   - *Abandonment is a form of neglect when the caregiver leaves the elderly person with no intention of resuming the caregiver role.*

   In the scenario, Pat's father is a victim of neglect and emotional abuse.

GROUP ACTIVITY

● PURPOSE OF THE ACTIVITY

The purpose of this activity is to examine the level of stress experienced during caregiving. The following activities can be completed as a class, in small groups, or individually.

Have the audience complete Handout 8-3. Include stress-reducing techniques in the discussion.

Name _____ Date _____

Program/Course _____ Instructor's Name _____

Caring for the Caregiver Pre- and Post-Test

1. Caregiving is stressful and labor-intensive. Persons who care for others experience more psychological and health-related problems. Symptoms of stress and depression are:
   a. Three times more common in caregivers when compared to noncaregivers.
   b. Ten times more common in caregivers when compared to noncaregivers.
   c. No different in caregivers when compared to noncaregivers.
   d. One hundred times more common in caregivers when compared to noncaregivers.

2. "Caregiver burden" is an industry term. What does it describe?
   a. The responsibility of watching a client 24 hours a day.
   b. The physical, emotional, financial, and social problems associated with caregiving.
   c. The lack of physical strength to care for debilitating clients and family members.
   d. The job of health care.

3. The signs and symptoms of caregiver burden can differ for each individual. The extent of symptoms depends on:
   a. The number of resources used by the client.
   b. The physical condition of the client or family member home.
   c. The personality, belief systems, general health, energy levels, and coping skills of the caregiver.
   d. The environment in which the caregiver works, as well as the amount of support given by other family members.

4. The most effective strategy to reduce the effects of caregiver burden and burnout is to manage the environment. List ways to manage the environment.
   a. Develop a plan and continually reevaluate the environment to reduce any unnecessary burdens.
   b. Incorporate support groups or regular case discussions into the plan.
   c. Discuss concerns with the supervisor or other members of the facility, family, friends, or physician.
   d. All of the above.

(continued)

Handout **8-1**

Caring for the Caregiver Pre- and Post-Test (Continued)

5. The stress of caring for the older adult is a significant risk factor for abuse and neglect. Chose from the following possible indicators of abuse from a caregiver:
   a. The caregiver or abuser may be apathetic or angry toward the elderly person.
   b. The caregiver or abuser may fail to assist the older adult with his or her needs.
   c. The caregiver or abuser may be noncompliant with service providers in planning for care.
   d. All of the above.

Common Signs of Burnout

Physical Signs	Psychological Signs	Behavioral Signs
Backaches	Anger and frustration	Emotional outbursts
Changes in eating habits	Decreased self-confidence and self-esteem	Withdrawal from friends and family
Elevated blood pressure	Loss of interest in hobbies and work	Loss of punctuality and neglect of duty
Fatigue	Feelings of inadequacy, helplessness	Decrease in judgment
Gastrointestinal problems	Feelings of restlessness	Inability to focus on tasks
Headaches	Depression	Tearfulness
Insomnia	Sense of being overwhelmed or overloaded	Increased use of chemical substances
Muscle tension	Mood swings	Difficulty getting along with others
Weight loss	Sense of failure	Impaired work performance
	Anxiety about future	Resistance to change

(O'Neill and McKinney, 2003)

Handout **8-2**

Caregiver Self-Assessment Questionnaire

During the past week or so, I have:	Yes	No
1. Had trouble keeping my mind on what I was doing.		
2. Felt that I couldn't leave my relative alone.		
3. Had difficulty making decisions.		
4. Felt completely overwhelmed.		
5. Felt useful and needed.		
6. Felt lonely.		
7. Been upset that my relative has changed so much from his or her former self.		
8. Felt a loss of privacy and/or personal time.		
9. Been edgy or irritable.		
10. Had sleep disturbed because of caring for my relative.		
11. Had a crying spell(s).		
12. Felt strained between work and family responsibilities.		
13. Had back pain.		
14. Felt ill (headaches, stomach problems, or the common cold).		
15. Been satisfied with the support my family has given me.		
16. Found my relative's living situation to be inconvenient or a barrier to care.		

17. On a scale of 1 to 10, with 1 being "not stressful" to 10 being "extremely stressful," please rate your current level of stress.	
18. On a scale of 1 to 10, with 1 being "very healthy" to 10 being "very ill," please rate your current health compared to what it was this time last year.	

Adapted from the Caregiver Self-Assessment Questionnaire (American Medical Association, 2006)

(continued)

Handout **8-3**

Caregiver Self-Assessment Questionnaire
(Continued)

How to Calculate Results

1. Count the number of *yes* responses for questions 1 through 4 and for question 16.

   Enter your total here: _____

2. Count the number of *no* responses for questions 5 through 15.

   Enter your total here: _____

   Total Score: _____

Scoring for Questions 1–16

The greater the Total Score, the higher the degree of stress being experience by the caregiver.

The caregiver is experiencing a high degree of distress if:

- A *YES* response was answered to either or both questions #4 and #11.
- The total score is 10 or more.

Scoring for Questions 17–18

Any rating 6 or higher indicates the Caregiver is experiencing a high degree of distress.

Adapted from the Caregiver Self-Assessment Questionnaire (American Medical Association, 2006)

Handout **8-3**

A Day in the Life of Pat: A Real-Life Scenario

Pat is a schoolteacher and has an elderly father with dementia. Since Pat's mom is deceased, the only option was to move Pat's father to live with Pat. Upon Pat's arrival home, water is flowing from the kitchen faucet, over the countertop, and onto the floor. Dad was found on the flooded kitchen floor, soiled. Pat becomes enraged and demoralizes him by yelling and screaming obscenities and insults.

1. List the possible causes for Pat's caregiver burden.

2. Describe the problem-solving approaches to help reduce caregiver burden.

3. Describe five types of abuse observed with the elderly. What types of abuse are noted in the scenario?

Handout **8-4**

MODULE 8
CARING FOR THE CAREGIVER

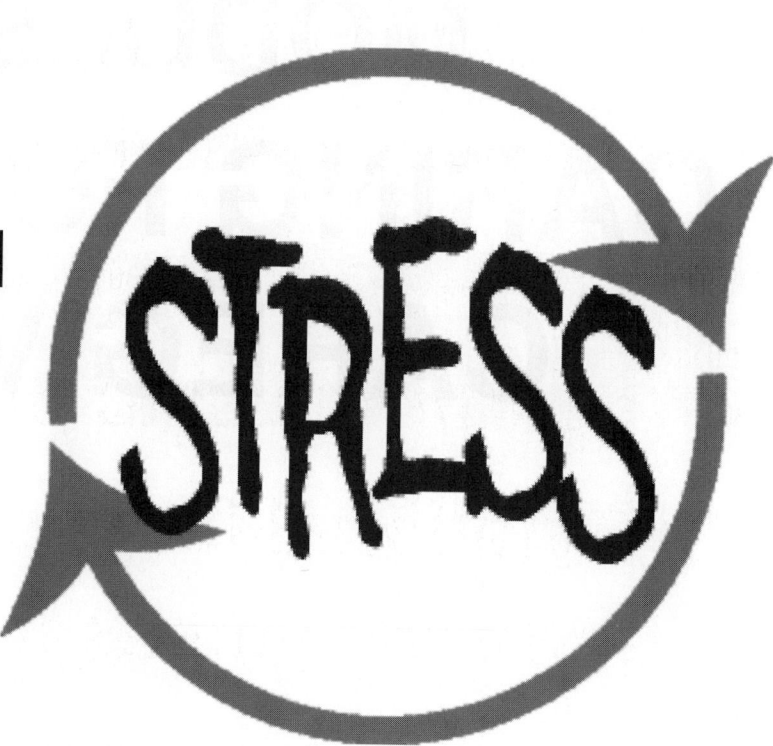

Causes of Caregiver Burden and Burnout

Physical

Emotional

Financial

Social

Informal Caregiver Burdens

- **Unexpected changes in role and social activities**
- **Physical demands (24/7)**
- **Learning basic nursing skills**
- **Emotional issues of a terminal illness**
- **Financial impact**

Formal Caregiver Burdens

- Includes informal caregiver burdens
- Lack of support from families and co-workers
- Workplace stressors

Needs of Clients in SNF

- **96.2% require assistance with bathing**
- **87.2% require assistance with dressing**
- **56.2% require assistance with toileting**
- **45% require assistance with eating**
- **25.4% require assistance with transfers**

STRESS

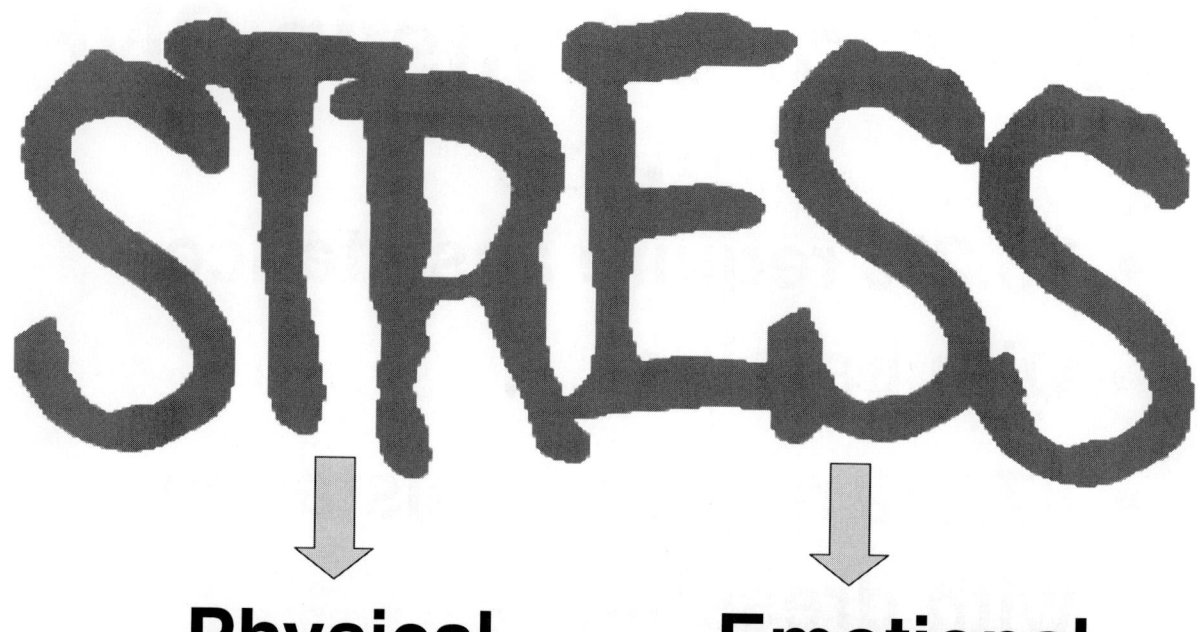

⬇ **Physical symptoms**   ⬇ **Emotional symptoms**

Problem Solving Approach

- **Define overall needs and goals**
- **Define problems**
- **Analyze strengths and weakness**
- **Determine resources**
- **Re-evaluate demands**

Problem Solving Approach (cont.)

- Set priorities
- Generate solutions
- Implement solutions
- Incorporate techniques to reduce stress
- Discuss concerns with the supervisor

Techniques to Reduce Stress

- **Time management skills**
- **Forget the super hero image**
- **Use relaxation techniques**
- **Exercise**

Techniques to Reduce Stress (*cont.*)

- Choose a favorite activity
- Talk to others
- Be flexible
- Healthy living

Healthy Living

- **Diet**
- **Rest**
- **Avoid tobacco**
- **Reducing risk factors**

Risk Factors

- **Non-modifiable = cannot be changed**

- **Modifiable = can be changed**

Elder Abuse

Categories of Elder Abuse

- **Domestic elder abuse**
- **Institutional elder abuse**
- **Self-neglect or self-abuse**

Types of Abuse

- **Physical abuse**
- **Emotional and physiological abuse**
- **Sexual abuse**
- **Financial abuse**
- **Neglect**
- **Abandonment**

Indicators of Abuse

- **Prevents the elder from speaking**
- **Apathy towards the elder**
- **Fails to assist or help**
- **Blames the elder**
- **Aggressive towards elder**

Indicators of Abuse (cont.)

- Overly affectionate around others
- Inappropriate sexual behavior
- Isolates the elder
- Contradictory versions
- Non-compliant with care
- Defensive

References

Module 1

ADEAR Alzheimer's Disease Education & Referral Center, A Service of the National Institute on Aging. Received via email: adear@alzheimers.org. Dated October 7, 2004.

National Institute on Aging. New prevalence study suggests dramatically rising numbers of people with Alzheimer's disease. Available at: http://www.nia.nih.gov/NewsAndEvents/PressReleases/PR20030818NewPrevalence.htm. Accessed November 6, 2004.

Rodgers AB. Alzheimer's disease: Unraveling the mystery. Alzheimer's Disease Education and Referral Center. Available at: http://www.alzheimers.org/unraveling/speak_kit.html. Accessed September 9, 2004.

Rovner BW, Folstein MF. Mini-mental state exam in clinical practice. *Hospital Practice*. 1987;22(1A):99,103,106,110.

Module 4

LeClerc CM, Wells DL. A feeding abilities assessment for persons with dementia. *Alzheimer's Care Quarterly*. 2004;5(2):123–134.

Module 5

Alzheimer's Association. 2006 National Public Policy Program to Conquer Alzheimer's Disease. Available at: http://www.alz.org/advocacy/2006program/5a.asp. Accessed June 6, 2006.

Camp C. *Montessori-Based Activities for Persons with Dementia*. (1999). Baltimore, MD: Health Professions Press; 1999.

Coyle J. Use it or lose it–do effortful mental activities protect against dementia? *New England Journal of Medicine*. 2003;348(25);2489–2490.

Flaherty G. Involving police when memory-impaired elders are missing. *Ageless Design*. Fall 2002;19. Available at: http://www.agelessdesign.com. Accessed March 13, 2005.

Warner M. (2002, Fall). Missing–what to do about wandering. *Advice and Advances Newsletter*. Ageless Design. Fall 2002, volume 19.

Zgola J. *Doing Things, A Guide to Programming Activities for Persons with Alzheimer's Disease and Related Disorders*. Baltimore, MD: The Johns Hopkins University Press; 1987.

Module 6

Merck Institute of Aging and Health. *The State of Aging and Health in America 2004.* Washington, DC: MIHA; 2004.

Reisberg B, Ferris SH, de Leon MJ, et al. The Global Deterioration Scale for assessment of primary degenerative dementia. *American Journal of Psychiatry.* September 1982;39(9):1136–1139.

Module 7

National Institute on Aging. New prevalence study suggests dramatically rising numbers of people with Alzheimer's disease. Available at: http://www.nia.nih.gov/NewsAndEvents/PressReleases/PR20030818NewPrevalence.htm. Accessed November 6, 2004.

Module 8

Administration on Aging. 2003 National Ombudsman reporting system data tables. Available at: http://www.aoa.gov/prof/aoaprog/elder_rights/LTCombudsman/National_and_State_Data/2003nors/2003nors.asp. Accessed April 20, 2005b.

American Medical Association, *Caregiver Self Assessment Questionnaire.* Available at: http://www.ama-assn.org/ama/pub/category/5037.html. Accessed May 16, 2006.

Bureau of Labor Statistics, U.S. Department of Labor. Personal and home care aides. *Occupational Outlook Handbook, 2004–05 Edition.* Available at: http://www.bls.gov/oco/ocos173.htm. Accessed April 20, 2005.

Bureau of Labor Statistics, U.S. Department of Labor. *Occupational Outlook Handbook, 2006–07 Edition, Personal and Home Care Aides.* Available at: http://www.bls.gov/oco/ocos173.htm. Accessed May 15, 2006.

National Association for Home Care & Hospice, *Basic Statistics about Home Care.* Available at: http://www.nahc.org/04HC_Stats.pdf. Accessed May 16, 2006.

National Family Caregiver Association, *National Family Caregivers Association (NFCA) Random Sample Survey of Family Caregivers, Summer 2000, Unpublished, on the internet at* http://www.thefamilycaregiver.org/who/stats.cfm#3 accessed May 15, 2006a.

O'Neill J, McKinney M. Care for the caregiver. Available at: http://hab.hrsa.gov/tools/palliative/chap20.html. Accessed April 20, 2005.

Resources

Web Sites

Alzheimer's Association
www.alz.org

Alzheimer's Disease Education & Referral Center (ADEAR)
www.alzheimers.org

ElderCare Online's Alzheimer's & Dementia Care Channel
http://www.ec-online.net/alzchannel.htm

Alzheimer*Support*.com
http://www.alzheimersupport.com

Brain explorer
http://www.Brainexplorer.org

Centers for Disease Control and Prevention (CDC)
http://www.cdc.gov

Coping with Caregiving with Jacqueline Marcell
www.wsradio.com/copingwithcaregiving

Dementia.com
www.dementia.com

Journal of Alzheimer's Disease
www.j-alz.com

National Alliance for Caregiving/Family Caregiver Alliance
www.caregiver.org

National Institute of Neurological Disorders and Stroke
www.ninds.nih.gov

The Forgetting: A Portrait of Alzheimer's (DVD also available)
http://www.pbs.org/theforgetting/

Additional Readings

Bridges BJ. *Therapeutic Caregiving: A Practical Guide for Caregivers of Persons with Alzheimer's and Other Dementia Causing Diseases.* 2nd ed. Seattle, WA: BJB Publishing; 1995.

Mace NL, Rabins PV. *The 36-Hour Day: A Family Guide to Caring for Persons with Alzheimer's Disease, Related Dementing Illnesses, and Memory Loss in Later Life.* Clayton, VIC: Warner Books; 2001.

Warner ML. *The Complete Guide to Alzheimer's-Proofing Your Home.* Rev. ed. Ashland, OH: Purdue University Press; 2000.

Answers to Pre- and Post-Tests

Module 1
a, c, b, b, a, c, a, b, d; see Slides 1-9 and 1-10 for answer to question 10.

Module 2
d, b, b, b, d

Module 3
b, b, d, d, d

Module 4
c, a, b, c, d

Module 5
d, a, b, d, b

Module 6
b, c, b, b, d

Module 7
d, b, c, a, a

Module 8
a, b, c, d, d

IMPORTANT! READ CAREFULLY: This End User License Agreement ("Agreement") sets forth the conditions by which Thomson Delmar Learning, a division of Thomson Learning Inc. ("Thomson") will make electronic access to the Thomson Delmar Learning-owned licensed content and associated media, software, documentation, printed materials, and electronic documentation contained in this package and/or made available to you via this product (the "Licensed Content"), available to you (the "End User"). BY CLICKING THE "I ACCEPT" BUTTON AND/OR OPENING THIS PACKAGE, YOU ACKNOWLEDGE THAT YOU HAVE READ ALL OF THE TERMS AND CONDITIONS, AND THAT YOU AGREE TO BE BOUND BY ITS TERMS, CONDITIONS, AND ALL APPLICABLE LAWS AND REGULATIONS GOVERNING THE USE OF THE LICENSED CONTENT.

1.0 SCOPE OF LICENSE

1.1 <u>Licensed Content.</u> The Licensed Content may contain portions of modifiable content ("Modifiable Content") and content which may not be modified or otherwise altered by the End User ("Non-Modifiable Content"). For purposes of this Agreement, Modifiable Content and Non-Modifiable Content may be collectively referred to herein as the "Licensed Content." All Licensed Content shall be considered Non-Modifiable Content, unless such Licensed Content is presented to the End User in a modifiable format and it is clearly indicated that modification of the Licensed Content is permitted.

1.2 Subject to the End User's compliance with the terms and conditions of this Agreement, Thomson Delmar Learning hereby grants the End User a nontransferable, nonexclusive, limited right to access and view a single copy of the Licensed Content on a single personal computer system for non-commercial, internal, personal use only. The End User shall not (i) reproduce, copy, modify (except in the case of Modifiable Content), distribute, display, transfer, sublicense, prepare derivative work(s) based on, sell, exchange, barter or transfer, rent, lease, loan, resell, or in any other manner exploit the Licensed Content; (ii) remove, obscure, or alter any notice of Thomson Delmar Learning's intellectual property rights present on or in the Licensed Content, including, but not limited to, copyright, trademark, and/or patent notices; or (iii) disassemble, decompile, translate, reverse engineer, or otherwise reduce the Licensed Content.

2.0 TERMINATION

2.1 Thomson Delmar Learning may at any time (without prejudice to its other rights or remedies) immediately terminate this Agreement and/or suspend access to some or all of the Licensed Content, in the event that the End User does not comply with any of the terms and conditions of this Agreement. In the event of such termination by Thomson Delmar Learning, the End User shall immediately return any and all copies of the Licensed Content to Thomson Delmar Learning.

3.0 PROPRIETARY RIGHTS

3.1 The End User acknowledges that Thomson Delmar Learning owns all rights, title and interest, including, but not limited to all copyright rights therein, in and to the Licensed Content, and that the End User shall not take any action inconsistent with such ownership. The Licensed Content is protected by U.S., Canadian and other applicable copyright laws and by international treaties, including the Berne Convention and the Universal Copyright Convention. Nothing contained in this Agreement shall be construed as granting the End User any ownership rights in or to the Licensed Content.

3.2 Thomson Delmar Learning reserves the right at any time to withdraw from the Licensed Content any item or part of an item for which it no longer retains the right to publish, or which it has reasonable grounds to believe infringes copyright or is defamatory, unlawful, or otherwise objectionable.

4.0 PROTECTION AND SECURITY

4.1 The End User shall use its best efforts and take all reasonable steps to safeguard its copy of the Licensed Content to ensure that no unauthorized reproduction, publication, disclosure, modification, or distribution of the Licensed Content, in whole or in part, is made. To the extent that the End User becomes aware of any such unauthorized use of the Licensed Content, the End User shall immediately notify Thomson Delmar Learning. Notification of such violations may be made by sending an e-mail to delmarhelp@thomson.com.

5.0 MISUSE OF THE LICENSED PRODUCT

5.1 In the event that the End User uses the Licensed Content in violation of this Agreement, Thomson Delmar Learning shall have the option of electing liquidated damages, which shall include all profits generated by the End User's use of the Licensed Content plus interest computed at the maximum rate permitted by law and all legal fees and other expenses incurred by Thomson Delmar Learning in enforcing its rights, plus penalties.

6.0 FEDERAL GOVERNMENT CLIENTS

6.1 Except as expressly authorized by Thomson Delmar Learning, Federal Government clients obtain only the rights specified in this Agreement and no other rights. The Government acknowledges that (i) all software and related documentation incorporated in the Licensed Content is existing commercial computer software within the meaning of FAR 27.405(b)(2); and (ii) all other data delivered in whatever form, is limited rights data within the meaning of FAR 27.401. The restrictions in this section are acceptable consistent with the Government's need for software and other data under this Agreement.

7.0 DISCLAIMER OF WARRANTIES AND LIABILITIES

7.1 Although Thomson Delmar Learning believes the Licensed Content be reliable, Thomson Delmar Learning does not guarantee or warrant (i) any information or materials contained in or produced by the Licensed Content (ii) the accuracy, completeness or reliability of the Licensed Content, or (iii) that the Licensed Content is free from errors or other material defects. THE LICENSED PRODUCT IS PROVIDED "AS IS," WITHOUT ANY WARRANT OF ANY KIND AND THOMSON DELMAR LEARNING DISCLAIMS AN AND ALL WARRANTIES, EXPRESSED OR IMPLIED, INCLUDING, WITH OUT LIMITATION, WARRANTIES OF MERCHANTABILITY OR FIT NESS OR A PARTICULAR PURPOSE. IN NO EVENT SHALL THOMSO DELMAR LEARNING BE LIABLE FOR: INDIRECT, SPECIAL, PUNITIV OR CONSEQUENTIAL DAMAGES INCLUDING FOR LOST PROFIT LOST DATA, OR OTHERWISE. IN NO EVENT SHALL THOMSON DELMA LEARNING'S AGGREGATE LIABILITY HEREUNDER, WHETHER ARI ING IN CONTRACT, TORT, STRICT LIABILITY OR OTHERWISE, EXCEE THE AMOUNT OF FEES PAID BY THE END USER HEREUNDER FO THE LICENSE OF THE LICENSED CONTENT.

8.0 GENERAL

8.1 <u>Entire Agreement</u>. This Agreement shall constitute the entire Agreement between the Parties and supercedes all prior Agreements and unde standings oral or written relating to the subject matter hereof.

8.2 <u>Enhancements/Modifications of Licensed Content</u>. From time t time, and in Thomson Delmar Learning's sole discretion, Thomson Delma Learning may advise the End User of updates, upgrades, enhancemen and/or improvements to the Licensed Content, and may permit the En User to access and use, subject to the terms and conditions of this Agree ment, such modifications, upon payment of prices as may be established b Thomson Delmar Learning.

8.3 <u>No Export</u>. The End User shall use the Licensed Content solely in th United States and shall not transfer or export, directly or indirectly, th Licensed Content outside the United States.

8.4 <u>Severability</u>. If any provision of this Agreement is invalid, illegal, o unenforceable under any applicable statute or rule of law, the provisio shall be deemed omitted to the extent that it is invalid, illegal, or unenforc able. In such a case, the remainder of the Agreement shall be construed i a manner as to give greatest effect to the original intention of the partie hereto.

8.5 <u>Waiver</u>. The waiver of any right or failure of either party to exercis in any respect any right provided in this Agreement in any instance sha not be deemed to be a waiver of such right in the future or a waiver of an other right under this Agreement.

8.6 <u>Choice of Law/Venue</u>. This Agreement shall be interpreted, con strued, and governed by and in accordance with the laws of the State of Nev York, applicable to contracts executed and to be wholly preformed therein without regard to its principles governing conflicts of law. Each party agree that any proceeding arising out of or relating to this Agreement or th breach or threatened breach of this Agreement may be commenced an prosecuted in a court in the State and County of New York. Each party con sents and submits to the nonexclusive personal jurisdiction of any court i the State and County of New York in respect of any such proceeding.

8.7 <u>Acknowledgment</u>. By opening this package and/or by accessing th Licensed Content on this Web site, THE END USER ACKNOWLEDGE: THAT IT HAS READ THIS AGREEMENT, UNDERSTANDS IT, AN AGREES TO BE BOUND BY ITS TERMS AND CONDITIONS. IF YOU D(NOT ACCEPT THESE TERMS AND CONDITIONS, YOU MUST NOT AC CESS THE LICENSED CONTENT AND RETURN THE LICENSED PROD UCT TO DELMAR LEARNING (WITHIN 30 CALENDAR DAYS OF THI END USER'S PURCHASE) WITH PROOF OF PAYMENT ACCEPTABLE T(THOMSON DELMAR LEARNING, FOR A CREDIT OR A REFUND. Shoul the End User have any questions/comments regarding this Agreemen please contact Thomson Delmar Learning at delmarhelp@thomson.com.